Review Copy

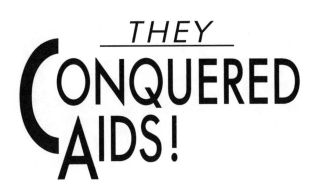

THEY
CONQUERED
AIDS!

THEY
CONQUERED
AIDS!

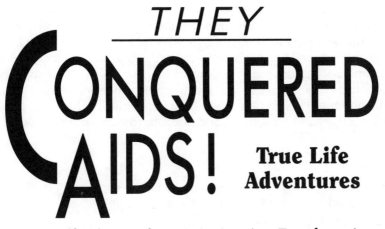

True Life
Adventures

From Self-Reliance, *thru* Inspiration, *into* Transformation

Scott J. Gregory, O.M.D.
Bianca Leonardo, N.M.D.

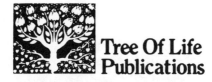

Tree Of Life
Publications

Disclaimer

The authors do not directly or indirectly dispense medical advice or prescribe any of the natural therapies for AIDS or any other illness. It is not the intent of the authors to diagnose or prescribe, but only to offer health information that the reader can consider, in cooperation with his chosen health specialist. In the event that you use this information without a health practitioner's approval, you are prescribing for yourself, which is your constitutional right, but the authors and publisher assume no responsibility.

Copyright © 1989 Tree of Life Publications

Tree of Life Publications: 255 N. El Cielo Rd., # 126
Palm Springs, CA 92262

Printed in the United States of America
First Printing March 1989
10 9 8 7 6 5 4 3 2 1

Library of Congress Cataloging-in-Publication Data

Gregory, Scott J.
    They Conquered AIDS! True Life Adventures: From
        Self-Reliance—Thru Inspiration—Into Transformation

    Includes Bibliography, Index
    1. AIDS (Disease)—Patients—United States—
Biography. 2. AIDS (Disease)—Alternative Treatment.
3. Holistic medicine. I. Leonardo, Bianca. II. Title.
RC607.A26G76   1989   616.97'9206   88-20135
ISBN 0-930852-03-6

DEDICATED

to Suffering Humanity

ACKNOWLEDGMENTS

We are grateful to all the health reformers and those who discovered and practiced the true healing arts, natural and spiritual, throughout the ages—many of whom suffered extreme persecution for their enlightened views: Hippocrates, Jesus, Paracelsus, Samuel Hanneman, Florence Nightingale, Mary Baker Eddy, Anna Kingsford, Isaac Jennings, Russell Trall, John H. Tilden, Herbert M. Shelton, John Harvey Kellogg, Norman Walker, and many others of former ages and our own, too numerous to mention. Special thanks to Dr. Alan Cantwell, Jr., for his foreword and his kindnesses, and all the other medical doctors who have crossed the line into the bright promise of holistic healing.

We thank the persons who shared their lives and gave us the interviews upon which this book is based; their medical and holistic doctors and helpers; Paul Herman Leonard, for his vital assistance; Mary Richardson, Al Gilbert, and others who helped the authors in the two years it took to bring this book to birth. May it bless all those in the world who are receptive to our message.

By the same authors:

CONQUERING AIDS NOW! With Natural Treatment, a Non-Drug Approach (a Warner Book)

Other books by Bianca Leonardo:

Cancer and Other Diseases Caused by Meat Consumption—Here's the Evidence

Deep Thoughts on War and Peace and Other Essays on the Vegetarian Way of Life

CONTENTS

Foreword by Alan Cantwell, Jr., M. D.

Photographs of the Conquerors

PART I

OVERVIEW:

THE CONQUERORS

(Brian Mitchell, Steven Greer, John Davies, Bertie Chapin, Paul Michael Allen, Charles Stevens and Wood are pseudonyms.)

PART II

    These true stories are a small sampling of Persons With AIDS who have conquered this dread disease. Their chosen paths were alternative, natural therapies and often a spiritual pursuit. There are many more such persons, but the media do not seek them out nor publicize them. Some of these persons do not want publicity. A few of the people interviewed wished to maintain their privacy, so pseudonyms were used. Their vital data is filed in the offices of the publisher. In the case of "Paul Michael Allen," it is filed in the office of the Hygeia Health Retreat.

    The opinions expressed in the personal accounts and commentaries in Part II not by the authors are the viewpoints of those writing and not necessarily the opinions of the authors.

Foreword

AIDS (acquired immune deficiency syndrome) is the most terrifying biological holocaust ever to appear on this planet. By 1991, it is predicted that 270,000 Americans will have contracted the deadly disease. In addition, hundreds of thousands of people will suffer from AIDS-related illnesses, and millions of other seemingly "healthy" people will be infected with the AIDS virus.

Currently, there is no good medical treatment for this "invariably fatal disease," nor is there a cure or a vaccine in the foreseeable future. The results of all this are too horrifying to contemplate.

The AIDS virus (originally known as "human T-cell leukemia/lymphoma virus-III" [HTLV-3], and now renamed "human immunodeficiency virus" [HIV]) is generally accepted as the "sole" cause of AIDS. Some scientists believe that the "origin" of the AIDS virus stems from an African green monkey virus that somehow "jumped" species into black Africans. From central Africa, the virus spread (in some unknown fashion) to the United States.

It was also theorized that the "mysterious" sexually-transmitted virus was picked up in Haiti by traveling New York City gays who brought the virus back to New York. From there, it was passed on to other gays. Recently, some AIDS "experts" have reversed the story. They claim New York City gays spread AIDS to Haiti.

We now know that the AIDS virus was first "introduced" into gay men in Manhattan (New York City) in late 1978. Proof of this is supplied by researchers who retrospectively tested old blood samples of young, primarily white Manhattan gays who volunteered as human guinea pigs for the government-sponsored hepatitis B vaccine trials that took place in Manhattan in November 1978. The trials continued through 1980. Testing of old (1978-1979) blood samples from these gay volunteers showed that almost 5% of the men carried antibodies to the AIDS virus at that time.

In January 1979, two months after the experimental vaccine trials began, the first AIDS case in a young Manhattan gay man was reported to the Centers for Disease Control (CDC). Additional hepatitis B vaccine trials using gays as experimental subjects began in March 1980 in Los Angeles, San Francisco, Denver, Chicago, and St. Louis. The first AIDS case from San Francisco was reported in the fall of 1980.

When the AIDS epidemic became "official" in the summer of 1981, the CDC reported the following data on the first 26 cases. All the cases were gay men. Twenty were from New York City: six were from Los Angeles and San Francisco. Twenty-five were white and one was black.

It is agreed now that AIDS is not a gay disease; heterosexuals—men and women (and also children)—have joined the group of Persons With AIDS.

Nevertheless, in a July 1987 *Playboy* report ("A Calm Look at AIDS"), AIDS experts like Robert Gallo (the co-discoverer of the AIDS virus) continue to stress that "AIDS will never become an overwhelming danger to the general public." In the same article Gallo also declared, "I personally don't know of a single case (in America) of a man getting the virus from a woman (through heterosexual intercourse)."

Despite these calming pronouncements, statistics show that AIDS is now the leading cause of death in young men and women in New York City, and one half-million New Yorkers are believed to be infected with the AIDS virus.

AIDS began in central Africa in the late 1970s—about the same time it began in New York City and in Haiti. We know that millions of blacks are infected, and that the disease in Africa is affecting men and women in equal numbers. The reason for this is not clear, but smallpox eradication vaccine programs sponsored by the World Health Organization during the late 1970s have been recently implicated in the spread of African AIDS. ("Smallpox Vaccine 'Triggered' AIDS Virus," *The London Times* May 11, 1987).

Experts believe that the vaccine program which inoculated over 90 million central African blacks with "Vacciniae virus" may have awakened a "dormant" AIDS virus infection in that population.

Unfortunately, most Americans still believe that AIDS is

a "gay" disease and that homosexuals are to blame for initiating and spreading the epidemic in America. There is still no satisfactory scientific explanation as to how a monkey virus out of Africa could have suddenly appeared and proliferated <u>exclusively</u> in the blood of young white gays in Manhattan. The profound significance of the question "why only gays?" should be pondered by all serious students of the AIDS epidemic.

On the basis of blood antibody studies, we know that the AIDS virus is "new." Although scientists claim that AIDS is a "new" disease caused by a new virus, it should be apparent that most AIDS illnesses and deaths are caused by Kaposi's sarcoma, *Pneumocystis carinii* pneumonia, tuberculosis, and opportunistic infections. <u>None of these diseases are "new."</u>

Kaposi's sarcoma (KS) is a form of cancer that was discovered more than a century ago in Vienna, Austria. Pneumocystis pneumonia, a lung infection due to a parasitic microbe, caused thousands of deaths in newborns and infant children in central Europe during the 1930s, 40s, and 50s. Mini-epidemics of Pneumocystis pneumonia have also occurred in U. S. hospitals, especially in children with cancer who are treated with immunosuppressive anti-cancer drugs.

Thus, it should be clear that other factors besides the AIDS virus must be operative to cause full blown AIDS.

Despite a decade of research and treatment in AIDS, the medical profession still is not clear as to exactly what AIDS is. Now that the experts know the AIDS virus is the "sole" cause of AIDS, the disease is technically no longer a "syndrome" but rather a disease caused by this specific virus.

One of the big problems in AIDS diagnosis is that each year there are bureaucratic changes in the official "definition" of what actually constitutes an "official" diagnosis of AIDS. For example, "dementia" due to AIDS virus brain infection is now accepted by the CDC as an "official" AIDS diagnosis. In 1987, it was also decided to include Tuberculosis infections (in patients who were AIDS antibody-positive) in the CDC definition of AIDS. The irony of all this is that thousands of people have already died of AIDS who did not fit (at the time) the official "definition" of AIDS. As a result, these deaths have not been included in the CDC AIDS statistics.

It should be obvious to all but the most naive investigators that AIDS-related complex (ARC) is AIDS. However, for CDC "statistical purposes" it is "classified" separately from AIDS. Many gay men have died from ARC but have not been counted as AIDS deaths.

What about a healthy person who tests "positive" for AIDS virus antibodies? Assuming that a "false-positive" reaction is ruled out, this is the earliest indication that the person has been exposed to the AIDS virus. However, by definition, this is not AIDS.

In the early stages of the epidemic, the experts believed that only a small percentage (about 10%) of "antibody-positive" persons would develop AIDS. By repeated antibody testing of large numbers of "positive" gay men, scientists now know that 50% (and possibly as many as 100%) of AIDS antibody "positive" reactors will eventually come down with AIDS or AIDS-related complex. The statistics are indeed depressing.

The AIDS virus is essentially a genetic package of death designed exclusively to target, attack, and destroy the immune system. In the sexual arena, everyone should take the necessary precautions to ensure that they do not acquire this virus, or pass it on to others. As a physician, I must disagree with the belief of Roger Walther (whose story you will read) that "if one is in good shape physically, he can resist any virus... no matter how it penetrates the body (because) the immune system should be able to handle it."

Needless to say, every sexually-active adult who enters a new sexual relationship in the 1980s (especially in cities like Los Angeles, New York and San Francisco) should practice "safe sex." Although there is no such thing as 100% absolute safe sex, the only real alternative is celibacy. Testing for AIDS antibodies is the only ethical choice for couples who wish to conceive.

What does the medical establishment have to offer persons newly diagnosed with ARC, AIDS, and those who test "positive?" The answer is "very little." This response should not be surprising in view of the fact that AIDS is invariably quoted as "always fatal."

Of course there is radiation for KS tumors, but this is not a "cure" for KS. And there are antibiotics of various sorts for

Pneumocystis pneumonia and other opportunistic infections. But at best, these drugs are only temporarily curative. In the long run, antibiotics simply are not effective in patients who have severely damaged immune systems.

There is little doubt that AIDS is a disease closely related to cancer. (Remember that the AIDS virus "family" includes viruses that are now linked to leukemia and lymphoma.) Sadly, after a century of cancer research, there is still no satisfactory treatment for most forms of cancer, and the half-million cancer deaths in America annually attest to that fact. And despite extensive research on the immune system, medical science has no drug that heals a damaged immune system.

What should a person do who has a "fatal disease" like AIDS?

People who have been exposed to the AIDS virus have few options. They can enter an "experimental" program and get a drug which is far more likely to harm them than to cure them, or they can take a drug like "AZT" which is the only FDA-approved drug available for AIDS patients—at the cost of $13,000 per year. The side effects of AZT are horrendous. About one-third of the already immunodepressed patients on this drug require blood transfusions due to the drug's toxicity.

Barring serious infections, many physicians who understand the futility of radiation and chemotherapy for AIDS, will now opt for <u>no treatment at all</u>. Often a patient is told to "come back when something else develops." With the passage of more time, cancer and severe opportunistic infections almost always occur.

The only other remaining option is taken primarily by courageous and adventuresome patients. And that option is to seek additional help and healing outside the medical establishment.

This choice makes many physicians angry for obvious reasons. They will tell you there are quacks and charlatans and all sorts of people who will harm you and prevent you from getting quality medical care. Of course, to some extent that can be true. If one is seriously ill with AIDS, one is almost always better off hospitalized under the care of a "team" of physicians trained in the emergency management of an AIDS crisis.

But assuming one is not in imminent danger of losing his

life, thoughtful persons in any stage of AIDS virus infection will seek counsel from persons who have improved their immune systems and who are "conquering" AIDS.

In my opinion, anyone who has survived a serious opportunistic AIDS infection (like Pneumocystis pneumonia or TB) for more than two years is experiencing some sort of "miracle." (Yes, I believe in miracles, and I believe God is alive and well.)

One of the best places to go for healing is to someone who has experienced a healing. There are people who have been close to death from AIDS, and who are now feeling well.

In this book by Gregory and Leonardo, you will read about people who are "conquering" AIDS. You should know that physicians tend to be highly skeptical of individual accounts of people who were hopeless cases and who found a way to heal themselves. Such stories are often pooh-poohed in medical circles as "anecdotes". Nevertheless, I must confess I enjoy reading about the experiences of people who have healed themselves of a life-threatening disease, like cancer or AIDS. And there is much to learn from their experiences.

Physicians, like any other group, have their peculiarities. I must admit I found myself bristling at some of the unorthodox ideas expressed in these stories by Persons With AIDS. Nevertheless, the stories are not meant to be "scientific." Rather, they document real life "do or die" agonizing struggles against the most deadly infectious disease of our time. As such, the individual experiences contained in these accounts of Persons With AIDS should serve well the needs of readers who are searching for alternative healing ideas and methods for conquering AIDS.

Time is of the essence. There is no doubt that a "crash course" in healing is essential for persons afflicted with AIDS! Even though this book is controversial, it is certainly filled with food for thought.

In terms of numbers, the male homosexual community in America is presently the group who is suffering most. I believe that through this painful collective experience, gay people will learn to serve as pioneer teachers and healers in the fight against AIDS. I am hopeful that through the power of love a higher healing consciousness will pervade the planet—and the epidemic will subside.

I wish I knew more about love, but I am only a student. However, there is a spiritual book that teaches a way to discover what love is, and I would like to recommend the book to those who are unfamiliar with it. It is called *A Course in Miracles*. Because AIDS now affects so many high-risk groups (gays, hemophiliacs, blacks, Hispanics, drug-addicts, prisoners, prostitutes) who are often unloved by society, I would like to quote a passage from "The Course" that explains, in part, what love is. I have found the words quite thought-provoking. It reads:

"Perhaps you think that different kinds of love are possible. Perhaps you think there is a kind of love for this, a kind of love for that; a way of loving one, another way of loving still another. Love is One. It has no separate parts or degrees; no kinds nor levels, no divergencies and no distinctions. It is like itself, unchanged throughout. It never alters with a person or a circumstance. It is the Heart of God, and also of His Son."

Alan Cantwell, Jr., M. D.
Los Angeles, CA
March, 1988

Dr. Alan Cantwell is a dermatologist and internationally known scientific researcher in the field of cancer and AIDS microbiology. He is also the author of the books *AIDS: The Mystery and the Solution,* (1984), and *AIDS and the Doctors of Death,* (1988). Both are published by Aries Rising Press, P.O. Box 29532, Los Angeles, CA 90029.

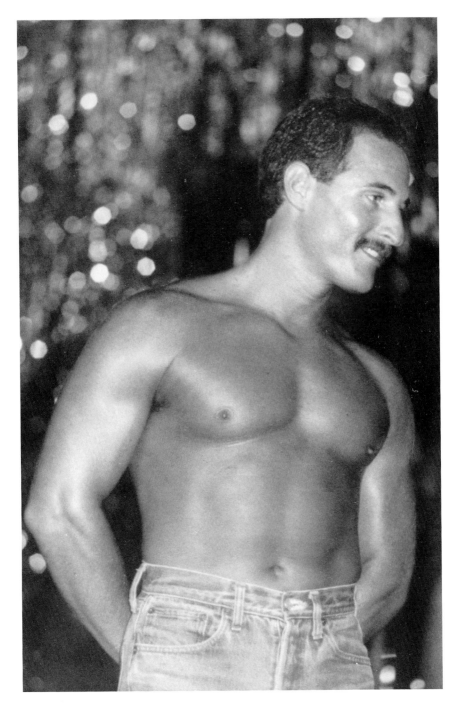

Louie Paul Nassaney

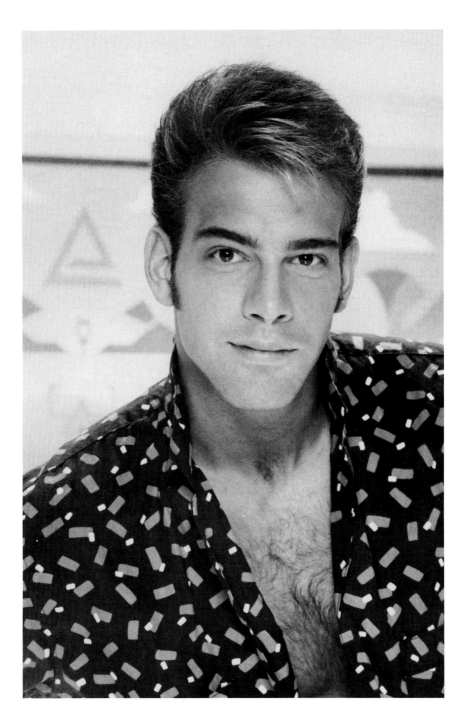

Russell John Carlton

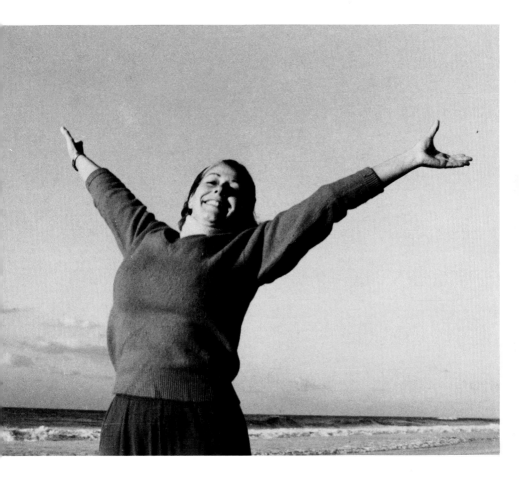

Niro Asistent

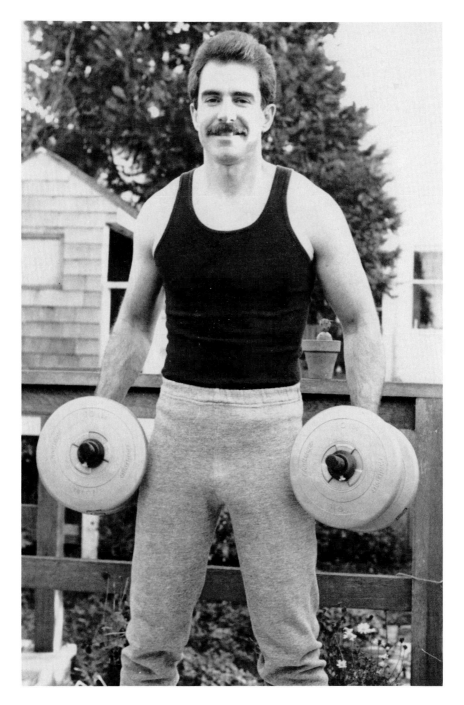

Daniel Turner
(Rink Foto, San Francisco)

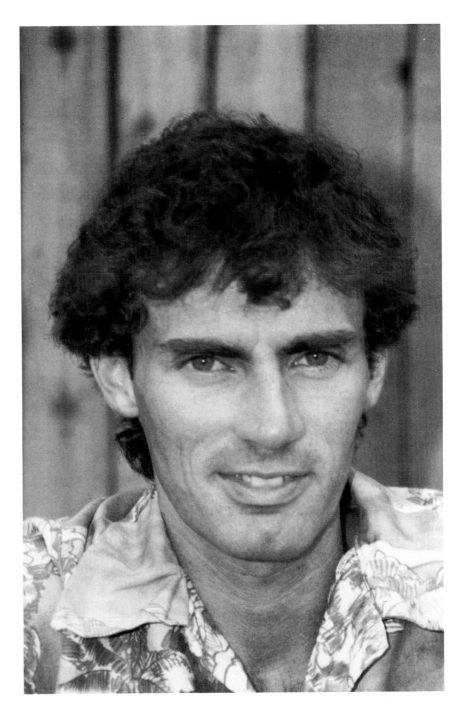

Tommy Griggs

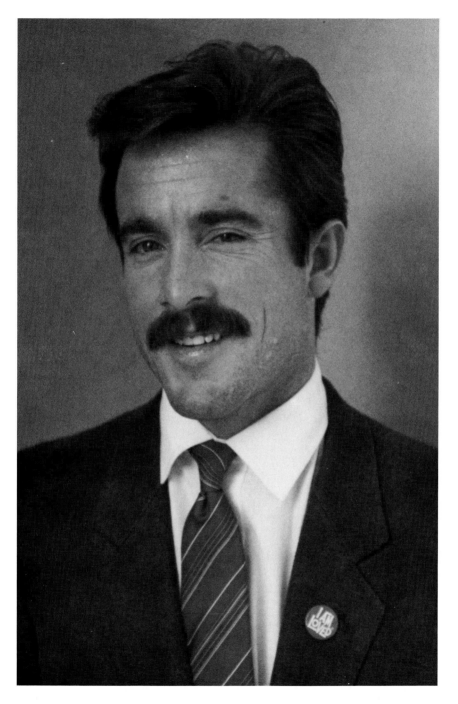

Douglas Johnson

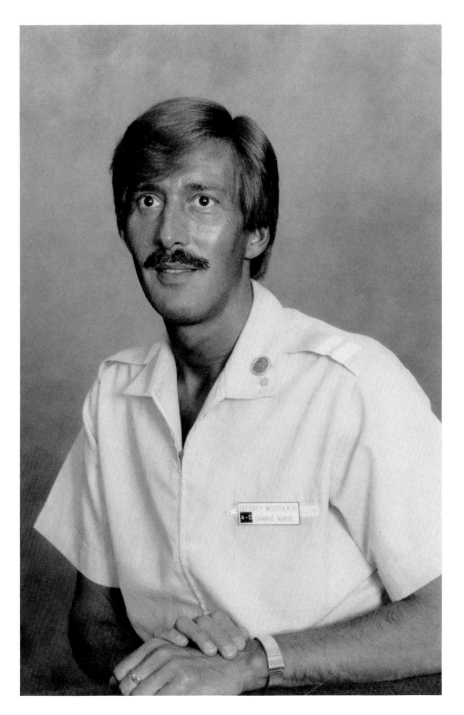

Jeffrey Joshua Migota, R.N.

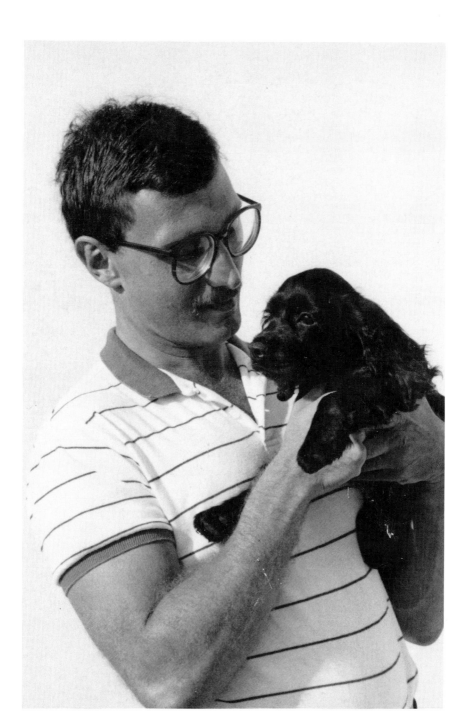

Roger Walther

Overview

TAKE CHARGE!

WORLDWIDE HEALING MODES

WHY NATURAL THERAPIES?

A-I-D-S OR X-Y-Z ?

TAKE CHARGE!

"Man alone is the architect of his destiny. The greatest revolution in our time is that human beings, by changing the inner attitudes of their minds, can change the outer aspects of their lives."

—William James, "Father of Psychology," 1902

For uncounted ages, the power of belief and faith—in good or evil—has been known by the religious mind. Now the scientists are coming forth to prove it.

Ernest Rossi, Ph.D., a clinical psychologist, Neuro-Linguistic programmer and renowned hypnotherapist, is the author of a book entitled *The Psychobiology of Mind-Body Healing.* In it, he offers study after study that point to the impact of belief systems on the causes and outcome of disease states. He opens with shocking, documented reports of tribal "voodoo death." A voodoo doctor points a bone at a designated victim, commands that he dies, and the victim succumbs to the imaginary power of the suggestion, usually within hours.

In addition, Dr. Rossi explores the average efficacy rates of placebos in 22 double blind studies. Patients consistently got pain relief evaluated at 56% (average) of the potency of powerful analgesics such as morphine and darvon—but all by sugar pills. The patients earnestly believed that these placebos were drugs and had power to relieve their pain, and so they did!

DO WE MAKE OURSELVES SICK?

We all have a divine and direct connection to the healing energies of the universe, and at any point in time that information and power are given to us all by simply asking.

Who knows your body better than you do? How long have you experienced messages of discomfort, such as disappointments, worry, fear, panic, pain, etc.? You can be free.

If you have trouble envisioning freedom, do some quick mental visualization. You have your mind with you at all times, and can do this wherever you are—without asking for help from others.

Think about a time in your life when you felt strong, powerful, healthy, happy—and watch how your body changes—especially your breathing and your posture. Listen to the "still, small voice within." It is a voice of inner guidance. It tells you where to go, who to see, or what you yourself must do to find that perfect balance with nature and the universe—including perfect health. Being in control exclusively makes you totally responsible and in control of your body and your mind. YOU ARE A WINNER! TAKE CHARGE AND MAKE THE DIFFERENCE! You create your own reality!

When you accept the idea that you have created what is in your life today, then you have taken responsibility and can change your experience and reality.

You can channel all your energy into what you believe in—whatever therapies feel right to you—that you feel an affinity for.

It is against freedom of conscious choice to be forced to take treatments in hospitals or elsewhere—treatments one does not believe in. We have all been victims in hospitals—from birth on.

The patient needs to overcome his passivity. People say to doctors, in essence: "Just do it to me. Give me a pill or a shot. Make me well. I take no responsibility." However, a few individuals today are learning a higher, more successful way to healing—and some of them are in this book.

We see highly vocal groups demonstrating, demanding that more federal money be spent on (useless) drug research for AIDS—without a single thought of how they could help themselves and the nation—by becoming responsible human beings, by TAKING CHARGE!

NEVER GIVE UP. No matter what you are looking for, you will find it, if you look hard enough.

The universe provides all. It loves you and wants you healthy and happy. You are a victorious, righteous conqueror. It is not someone else's faith, but yours, that can make you well. Feel it! Ask, search, seek out, and help conquer AIDS now! TAKE CHARGE!

WORLDWIDE HEALING MODES

Primitive or original medicine, today called "folk medicine," was the antecedent of all medicine.

ORIENTAL MEDICINE

Chinese medicine is at least 2,500 years old. One of its principal therapies is acupuncture. Its major premise is that there are channels called meridians throughout the body that store energy. The acupuncture needle is inserted in the body, and often, after a few minutes of treatment, pain is relieved. However, this is not its only purpose. Most diseases that are treated by Western medicine can be also treated by Chinese medicine. In some cases, acupuncture alone is used, in some cases herbs, and in others, both together. Western medicine is superior in certain cases, especially in emergencies. There are many uses for acupuncture: as anesthesia, in emergency situations (such as reviving consciousness in cases of drowning, heat exhaustion, sunstroke, convulsions, shock, and coma), in the treatment of all kinds of diseases, in obstetrics, and for conditions of the eye, ear, nose, and throat. It is not generally understood how acupuncture works, although there are many theories—but it is obvious that it does work.

In Oriental Medicine, herbs are understood and widely used. Moxibustion is a therapy in which herbs and acupuncture are used together. Indirect moxibustion: the practitioner takes a stick made of the herb moxa, burns the end, which lights up like a cigar, and holds the glowing tip an inch or so above various acupuncture points, thereby stimulating them. Direct moxibustion: the pure moxa plant is used and rolled in long thin cords which are heated, made into tiny balls, then applied to acupuncture points. Just prior to scarring the skin, the hot moxa is removed.

Acupuncture has five basic uses: (1) pain control, sedation, anesthesia; (2) energy movement (adding or lessening it); (3) treatment of organs; (4) tonification; and (5) wrinkle removal.

When materials get clogged in a river, a blockage is created. The river is stagnant; there is a stoppage of its flow. So it is with the body. When sickness occurs, the channels are blocked. To unblock the channels, the acupuncture needle is used.

Cupping is another form of treatment. The practitioner takes an acupuncture needle and inserts it into a meridian point. Then a heated glass or bamboo cup is put over the area creating suction which removes stagnant blood. A special type of massage uses the bowl of a spoon to get this same result.

Acupuncture was licensed in the U.S. in 1970, after President Nixon visited the People's Republic of China and established relations with that country.

It is such a new healing modality that as of 1988, there are only 6,000 acupuncturists in the U.S. nationwide.

AYURVEDA IN INDIA

In India, a healing method is known as Ayurveda. It is evolved from the Vedas, the ancient sacred literature of Hinduism calculated to be about 4,000 years old, and is still used in India. What is Ayurveda? Literally it means "The Science of Life," (Ayur = life, Veda = science). This traditional Indian system of medicine covers both the knowledge of life and the knowledge of healthy living. Ayurvedic techniques are not only ancient, but revolutionary within the context of preventive medicine. Ayurveda is said to go far beyond healing and prevention. It is an approach to immortality and to ultimate enlightenment by achieving a lively presence of the unified field in the body, mind, and consciousness.

Charaka, in the second century A. D., was one of the great names in Ayurveda. He composed an encyclopedia of medicine which is still used in India and gave to his followers an almost Hippocratic conception of their calling—"not for self, not for the fulfillment of any earthly desire of man, but solely for the good of suffering humanity should you treat your patients and so excel all."

WESTERN MEDICINE

Western medicine began in Egypt and proceeded to Greece. Hippocrates, a celebrated physician of Greece (400 B.C.), is regarded as the Father of Medicine. However, there is little similarity between his methods and those of Western Medicine in the twentieth century, and the changes are not always to mankind's benefit. His "Hippocratic Oath" is a basis for medical ethics and is taken by students about to receive the M.D. degree, even today. But its demands are diluted. The code demands: "First do no harm." Oh, that the doctors of the twentieth century would follow this command!

Hippocrates said that the body basically heals itself when allowed. This belief is a basic tenet of holistic healing. He declared that disturbances such as fevers and colds appear in the body where healing is happening, and these are "renormalization" processes. The body is "cleaning house" and should be left alone to do its work. Nature and the body have a "wisdom" that should be listened to; mankind should not immediately rush in with medical interference for every problem. This extreme dependence upon the huge medical complex is good for the income of the medical personnel involved, but often bad for the health of the sick individual.

The holistic healing movement of today agrees with many of the ancient concepts. But the drugs used by Western Medicine for every possible symptom merely suppress these symptoms and never get at the cause. They simply accumulate in the body, and often create a greater problem later.

Here is a shocking statistic: there are about 350,000 over-the-counter medications on the market in the U.S., reports Dr. Gregg Warshaw of the American Academy of Family Physicians. Americans spend an estimated $4,000,000,000 to $5,000,000,000 (billion dollars) on those medications every year. We are a nation of drug addicts. The overuse of legal drugs inevitably leads to the illegal ones—of course not in all individual cases—but this is true as a national trend.

Hippocrates said: "Let food be thy medicine." This statement refers directly to that large area of health called nutrition, and while today there is much interest in the subject, wholesome foods are not considered to be capable of acting as medicines to the vast majority of mankind. Yet, it is a fact that there are persons who, with proper nutrition and other natural elements, maintain their health and never need the services of physicians or use drugs.

Aristotle (300 B.C.), who was not a doctor but a philosopher, believed that disease is identifiable by certain symptoms, and most important in the diagnosis of disease was to name it. The theory was that physical manifestations needed to be altered physically. If it offends, cut it out! Thus began the harsh practice of surgery, often unneeded.

Aristotle's philosophy is what dominates modern medical theory and practice. Today we have chemical drugs in addition. The body is considered to be a machine. So much so, that today modern surgery gives the body/machine replaceable parts, as with an automobile.

Today's natural therapies return to the correct doctrines of Hippocrates, the Father of Medicine.

Galen was a Greek physician and writer (130-200 A.D.). He wrote about medicine, but made many errors. Dissection was forbidden in Greek culture, which resulted in a number of mistakes in the field of anatomy; e.g., Galen declared that the anatomy of a pig and a man are identical, which is not so.

Paracelsus, Swiss-born alchemist and physician, reintroduced Hippocratean research in the 1500s.

Errors—medical and others—are perpetuated for hundreds, even thousands of years! Medical doctors in our century are following Aristotle of ancient Greece in an era over 2,000 years ago,—and he was wrong.

We are reminded of the infamous case of Louis XIV in the field of childbirth. In France in the 1600s—300 years ago, women always gave birth on "birthing stools" with the help of female midwives. Louis had many wives and mistresses who gave birth in the palace. He liked to view the process, but could see little when the woman, greatly covered, was laboring to give birth on a stool. So he devised a way that he could see everything—from behind a curtain. He convinced his court that it would be better for the birthing women to lie flat on a table and have doctors or male midwives attend them. Stirrups to lift the legs high were added. This made it very convenient for the king to see everything, by peeking from behind curtains at the babies being born, but much more difficult for the birthing mother, who no longer had gravity to work with her in labor.

So started the monstrous error of putting the laboring mother in this totally wrong and unnatural position. From the practice at the court, it spread all over the nation, and to Europe and America. It is still being practiced—and so the medical establishment is "married to a mistake"—following the whim of a foolish and arrogant king 300 years ago! Isn't that incredible?[1]

In the U.S. in the 1800s, Samuel Hahneman, "father of homeopathy", reintroduced the concepts of Hippocrates. He realized that bleeding people made them worse; in fact, it often killed them. George Washington was one of the victims of this stupid and cruel practice.

Homeopathy[2] is becoming more popular today, both in the United States and Europe. Britain's royal family entrusts its health to this controversial holistic healing art, which claims to boost the immune system.

---

[1]   Arms, Suzanne. *Immaculate Deception — A New Look at Women and Childbirth*, page 24, Bantam Books, 1977. (Recommended reading as a study in childbirth in our time. A passionate, fully-documented examination of the myths and realities of childbirth.)

[2]   More on Homeopathy: "In an 1890 issue of Harper's Magazine, Mark Twain observed that the then thriving practice of homeopathic medicine had 'forced the old school doctor to stir around and

In 1847, the American Medical Association was formed. It molded the medical theory and practice in the U.S., now based largely on drugs and surgery for correction and on the mechanical concept of man—rather than on natural healing, with herbs, nutrition and prevention. It disregarded the Hippocratean doctrine that the body can heal itself, with some gentle help from harmless and natural methods and therapies, such as fresh air, sunshine, water, exercise, wholesome foods, herbs, sleep and rest, quietness, kindness, positive thinking, peace of mind, etc. By going back to the pristine purity of natural and spiritual living—mankind can prevent disease! But it has largely forgotten the natural and spiritual in health matters.

In the 140 years since the A.M.A was formed, the billion-dollar drug complex has come into being. It's a huge Frankenstein of a monster, and untold sins are being committed in its name. Very often, the profit to be made with drugs is more important than the welfare of the patient. Today's "health care" is the branch of the tree of healing that has become malignant. It is not "health care" so much as "disease care." True

---

²Continued

learn something of a rational nature about his business.' At the time, homeopathy was a respected branch of medical science, taught in 22 homeopathic medical schools, and practiced by 15 percent of U.S. physicians. Now, gaining new popularity through its claim of being a natural way to boost the body's defense system, this controversial 200-year-old healing system may once again force the medical establishment to 'stir around' and reexamine some of its basic assumptions about fighting disease.

"Based on principles developed in the late 1700s by German physician Samuel Hahnemann (1755-1843), homeopathy — with its twin principles of 'like cures like' and 'less is more' — stands in marked contrast to today's conventional, or allopathic, approach to health, which often seems preoccupied with counteracting merely the symptoms of disease. And while even proponents will concede health care would include the teaching of prevention to a much larger degree.

Let us give credit where it is due. Some marvels are accomplished, certainly in cases of accidents and other crises, but as for healing the sick, Western medicine is on the wrong track. Drugs do not heal the sick; they only suppress symptoms.

The medical profession believes and claims that drugs do no harm. Their training causes them to "wear blinders" to the true facts.

Listening to their doctors causes people to mirror the same belief and faith in drugs, to their detriment.

The worst aspect of drugs is that they poison the body, and all have side effects. They are simply substances that do not belong in the body! Drugs often cause the symptoms to vanish, but that is a poor bargain to make with them. At a later time, other problems occur, or the same ones reoccur—and the drugs are not seen or accused as the cause.

Older citizens especially are overmedicated. Nearly 80% of people 65 and older have at least one chronic condition; about one-third have three or more. To combat their problems,

---

2 continued

> that some of homeopathy's concepts seem to defy the laws of science as we know them, they argue that results are what matter. Results are apparently why it has won and kept such influential adherents as Britain's royal family and, proponents say, help explain why it has been seen as a threat to be eradicated by the medical and pharmaceutical establishment.
>
> "Supporters are now looking to the role homeopathy will play in treating what appear to be the chronic diseases of the future, diseases against which the machines and chemicals of allopathic medicine have so far been largely ineffective."
>
> (From article "Royal Medicine," *New Age Journal*, Sept./Oct. 1987, pages 45-47, based on Dana Ullman's book *Homeopathy: Medicine for the 21st Century*.)

they rely on a battery of over-the-counter and prescription drugs, the majority of them using more than five medications (10% take more than twelve!) Effects: interactions among drugs and too great a quantity cause a host of complications, from mental confusion to slowed blood clotting to disturbance of the heart's rhythm.

There are innumerable people in the U.S. who have suffered much at the hands of today's Medicine—losing life, limb, and sometimes going into deep debt. We hear of persons who have lost their homes as a result of their huge medical bills and are living in the streets. Yet they did not regain their health. Is this " the American Way" of freedom, health, and abundance?

Natural therapies are not only safe but economical. This is a time when the huge medical bills of AIDS patients and others threaten to bankrupt the insurance companies, and perhaps the U.S. Here is another reason why natural therapies should be given widespread attention and tried.

Dr. Benjamin Rush, signer of the Declaration of Independence and well-known physician of the Colonial era, declared against medical monopolies, and an official recognition of any one system of medicine. Although the framers of our nation's documents forbade the establishment of a state religion, Dr. Rush's opposition to a state-blessed system of medicine, unfortunately did not make it into our great national documents. The result, 200 years later, is a medical monopoly, a drug despotism, and a collusion amongst the greatest powers of the nation: government, the media, the medical establishment, the university research centers, and the drug companies. This is exactly what Dr. Rush would have wanted to outlaw. We have freedoms in so many areas of life, but not freedom in matters of health and life.

In 1934, the A.M.A. House of Delegates adopted these principles of monopoly: "All features of medical service in any method of medical practice should be under the control of the medical profession. No other body or individual is legally or educationally equipped to exercise such control."

Monopoly is un-American, yet the medical profession wants a monopoly in disease and health care. It almost has it, through the sheer force of its money and power. Americans, and especially Congress, should open their eyes to this infringement on freedom in the United States.

Any change in health practices is considered a threat to the medical profession. Dr. Raymond Keith Brown, M.D., states: "Much of today's medical turmoil results from the medical establishment's resistance to change."

Alan Gregg, M.D., states: "Orthodoxy must pay a penalty, like a parking ticket, for staying too long in the same place."

The non-conformist doctors, trying to humanize medicine with some of the holistic health practices, are persecuted by their own organization, the A.M.A. And the F.D.A. does the same. In 1906 the Pure Food and Drug Act was passed, and then the Food and Drug Administration was founded. Its business is to see to it that the public has pure food and drugs— but it has gone far beyond the original intent. Now, protected by its government status, it persecutes and prosecutes non-conformist practitioners.

Yet there is hope. There is a small but growing number of enlightened medical doctors today who see the faults and limitations of the orthodox methods, and are protesting them. They have adopted holistic therapies, the teaching of prevention and nutrition, and some type of spiritual approach. Among them are: Drs. Stuart M. Berger, William G. Crook, Michael Klaper, John A. McDougall, Anthony J. Sattilaro, Bernie S. Siegel, Carl Simonton, Lendon Smith, Jonathan Wright, and others.

In the San Francisco area, there is a group called Meta-Physicians—physicians dedicated to bringing spiritual consciousness into the healing practice. This is very encouraging.[1]

There are a number of problems with allopathic medicine. More people are coming to the conclusion that often medical doctors cannot heal their patients. AIDS is today's flagrant example of doctors' helplessness and mankind's doubt and despair. No drug is on hand that can assure a healing, nor can a vaccine be found to cure AIDS. The reason is: how can diseased bodies—in many cases already polluted with too many drugs—be healed by adding another drug? The body must be purified to be healed. Drugs can suppress symptoms, but they cannot heal.

There is a great deal of guesswork—not only in the AIDS crisis—but in all of medicine. There are too many variables. The diagnosis of the doctor could be wrong; the laboratory results could be in error; the patient could misinform the doctor; there are many thousands of drugs—far too many for anyone to understand them all—especially their side effects. And, above all, there is allopathic medicine's basic and erroneous premise that man is merely a material body which needs to be treated with material medicines.

The mind is a powerful force, its influence great but very subtle and largely unknown. The power of the mind cannot be measured in a laboratory or a hospital. There, only physical causes and effects are considered.

NATURAL HYGIENE

Natural Hygiene is one of the modern schools of disease prevention and healing. It started in the United States about 100 years ago; there is renewed interest in it today. "Hygiene" does not mean cleanliness here. Its fundamental meaning is "the science of health and its maintenance." (Webster.) The

---

[1] MetaPhysicians—Terry Tyler, M.D., 2309 Eunice, Berkeley, CA 94708, Tel: 415/524-2165.

Greek goddess of health was named Hygeia.

A number of enlightened medical doctors were the pioneers in this movement of natural methods— Drs. Trall, Tilden, Kellogg, and Shelton.

These are its basic principles: (1) A vegetarian diet, much of it fruits and vegetables uncooked. (2) Autointoxication as the principal cause of disease: the body poisons itself with harmful substances and practices. (3) The body can cleanse itself of toxins and cure itself of disorders by fasting.

SPIRITUAL HEALING

Spiritual healing and spiritual science are other areas that should be investigated. The progenitor for our day's "New Age" varied spiritual paths was Mary Baker Eddy (1816-1910). She presented to the world a totally spiritual method of healing. A religious age interpreted her method as a religion, manifesting as a church. But the truth of the matter is that it is a spiritual science, and is valid in all ages.

In this latter part of the twentieth century, there are many spiritual paths. Some of today's spiritual paths have been explored by our Persons Who Have Conquered AIDS. Introductory material is also presented in Part II of this book.

WHY NATURAL THERAPIES?

Natural therapies should be given a greater opportunity to reach the people. Indeed, many Persons With AIDS—disillusioned with the medical system—have found the answers to their health problems in Holistic Healing. Some of these people were interviewed for this book.

Some Benefits of Natural Therapies

(A) Natural therapies improve the quality of life. They are safe, harmless, and effective. Their effectiveness depends partly on the devotion of the patient in using them and his faith in them and in himself. Patience is always involved. It takes a while for a body to get sick, and it often takes a while to recover under natural methods.

(B) Natural therapies increase the life expectancy of patients, compared with those taking drugs.

(C) The modalities prove effective in terms of T-cell function, the increase of immunity, changes in the blood chemistry, the restoration of energy, etc. Specific combinations of natural treatments work together; they are cumulative in their effects. There are at least twenty modalities that Holistic Healing has to offer.[1]

(D) The patient is involved in his own healing. Natural and spiritual therapies and treatments change the character of the patient in many ways. He takes responsibility; he decides or helps decide what should be done, how the treatment should proceed. He is not totally at the mercy of another's decisions.

---

[1] See the introductory material in *Conquering AIDS Now!* by the authors.

After his holistic healing, the patient has more knowledge on how to stay healthy, with nutrition and natural care of the body. He has educated himself in healing processes and preventive methods.

The Obstacles to a Wide Acceptance of Natural Therapies

(A) The medical establishment has not tested them. Why not? Because the avenues for research are closed. The basic premise for cure in the medical system is diametrically opposed to that in natural therapy systems.

There has been no federal funding to test methods of holistic healing.

Government agencies and foundations are not interested in natural health education and treatment. Alternatives interfere with standard methods and could mean great financial losses for the medical complex if cures were found for the major diseases. Organizations receiving untold sums of money would no longer profit. (A 1988 report states that AIDS is adding at least $15,000,000,000 [billion dollars] additional profits annually to the drug/medical coffers.)

There is a lack of support from foundations, government agencies, research project groups—all of whom conduct testing and disseminate information. Billions of dollars are being poured into these channels. The major media present only what is fed to them by the establishment.

There is big money in selling drugs to patients. There is no money in healing people with natural therapies such as fresh air, sunshine, water, and proper food, and little money in acupuncture, massage, supplying herbs and supplements, or in teaching people how to live a healthy lifestyle.

(B) Belief systems. Medical colleges are supported by the billion-dollar drug complex. Hence, students are taught what the drug companies want them to learn: namely, that diseases are to be treated with drugs. But the medical students are not advised that all drugs have dangerous side effects. Medical students are taught theories: the germ theory, the theory of immunization, the theory of pasteurization, etc. These theories are part of doctors' training, later to appear in their treatments. But these theories, and others, are only part of their originators' belief systems.

(C) There's a disbelief that natural therapies work. Medical propaganda and the media claim that drugs are the only way to health and to relieve pain. But, in the world of holistic medicine, acupuncture and herbs are found to be harmless and effective ways to abolish pain, without side effects. There are other natural methods also.

Most people will only take or do something upon their doctors' recommendations (called "doctor's orders".)

(D) There is much professional jealousy among doctors. Most researchers are trying to discover something new, hold it back, keep it confidential, or get personal credit. Some also discredit their associates.

(E) The results of natural therapies are difficult to measure, and are more subjective. (One cannot touch, feel, see or test them.) Medical protocol is more objective. Clinical laboratory data, verifiable T-cell ratio function, positive HIV— all these have nothing to do with the mental, psychological or spiritual state of the individual. But these states have a profound effect on health and the healing process.

(F) Disinterest. The majority of people are not interested in investigating new therapies. They are in a passive state, a "do it to me—you cure me" consciousness. They take little or no responsibility themselves, either in prevention or cure. They have been trained by the medical profession to expect doctors to give pills and inject them with drugs.

(G) There is a blackout of information on natural therapies by a powerful combine of the medical-pharmaceutical complex, the government, research departments of the universities, the media, etc.

(H) The medical establishment makes the rules. For example: when symptoms such as those in AIDS vanish, the patient looks and feels well, his tests substantiate his belief that he is well, yet the medical doctor calls it a remission (liable to return). Why cannot we say that the patient is well? Because the medical establishment makes the rules, and now the rule is this: no one can say he has conquered AIDS until 15 years have gone by. New rules are being made constantly.

In this book, we are making our own rules—and claiming that the individuals interviewed have conquered AIDS.

(I) Medical Requirements: These are the requirements the medical establishment sets for a documented cure of AIDS: the patient's blood chemistry must show a negative HIV; the helper T-cells must be normal; the suppressor T-cells normal; the subset ratio normal; and all tests must show normal T-cell function; all signs and symptoms related to AIDS or ARC must be gone. In accordance with this—how can the natural healer and his patients possibly come up with all these requirements? For example: a patient has had natural treatments, the symptoms are gone, he looks and feels fine, but all the above are not verified, so his healing is not believed.

Why the Public Does Not Hear About Cases of AIDS Healings, Although People Are Recovering

The general consensus in the medical community and hence in the public mind is that AIDS is an invariably fatal disease. This opinion must be changed. There are recoveries!

Groups for Persons With AIDS (PWAs) exist. How about a new group for PWHAs—Persons who HAD AIDS? It would certainly be elite. These "recoverees" are small in number and scattered all over the country.[1]

It is a worldwide belief that all AIDS victims die. A healing with natural therapies contradicts this belief. Very few persons want to be part of a group that goes against the general consensus of public opinion. When a person knows something unorthodox that is helpful to himself, he often does not want to share it with others, because it is dangerously different from the norm.

Some natural healers claim success with AIDS, but when it comes to actual verification, deterrent factors may come into play, especially two: the healer has lost touch with the patient or the patient desires to remain anonymous.

Other problems face a natural healer. The patient usually turns to natural therapies as a last resort, but often wants to keep "one foot" in the other camp and take drugs also. The patient wavers in his trust, not having lived in the natural way previously. There may be complications in the diagnosis procedures, lack of agreement about the symptoms, inaccurate tests, and the problem of interpretation.

---

[1] After constant declarations that AIDS is invariably fatal, this news item appeared: "A Medical Mystery—Researchers Hunt for the Longest-Surviving AIDS Patients." The article refers to "two men who could still be alive even though they may have been infected with the deadly virus as early as 1974. Both men are believed to be living somewhere in New York City. If scientists can find them and they agree to cooperate, the researchers hope to learn why they have been able to survive so long. This information could help others infected with the disease, which usually destroys the immune system." (*Los Angeles Times*, March 28, 1988. Article by Rob Stein.)

(Dear Establishment: Please read this book—*THEY CON-QUERED AIDS!* —and you will discover many more than two persons who have recovered, and learn some vital new facts on how it is possible to conquer AIDS!)

There is panic and fear, a feeling of haste for a healing, a belief that time is running out, etc. So the role of a natural healer in the case of an AIDS patient is not an easy one.

AIDS is a very personal and touchy subject. It deals with sexual preferences, lifestyle habits such as visiting prostitutes, drug abuse and addiction, or the illness of hemophilia. A patient is asked personal information, but may not wish to give it.

AIDS patients sometimes go into a panic and return to drug treatments. The vast majority of patients are taking orthodox medical treatments, and many individuals want to be part of the majority.

AIDS is partly a fear-induced disease, and the terror of catching AIDS is a subject that deserves more attention. A new epidemic of fear, which one doctor calls "FRAIDS," is widespread in the U.S. and elsewhere.

Upon receiving a diagnosis of AIDS, some individuals feel actually relieved. They no longer have to live with the anxiety of contracting AIDS. In some cases, these persons feel that for the first time in their lives, they are a part of something, part of a group with AIDS. There is a feeling of closeness, a sharing, a common bond—of impending tragedy, with life and death in the balance.

There is fear, but also an excitement. It's like living "on the edge," not knowing what is going to happen, not knowing if one is going to die tomorrow. Having AIDS puts the individual into an accelerated mental state. In some ways, it brings a new identity. When gay men meet each other, opening remarks usually include: "Are you HIV positive?"

Ironically, AIDS—which has already brought so much death—has also proved to be a way to bring people closer together, in a new commonality of shared danger and love.

The people who have recovered from AIDS decided they need not die for lack of a "miracle vaccine". They were not willing to accept the death sentence because there is no medical cure. The "recoverees" are definitely in the minority; most of the Persons With AIDS under medical treatment do die.

The medical establishment is disinterested in hearing about natural healings because they are clearly not the result of medical treatments. Self-healing, learning to become your own physician, is an anathema to the medical profession.

New Paths, New Hope

The healings in this book are interesting but not sensational. The people used no one method, but each selected his own non-medical path—natural and sometimes spiritual.

The "recoverees" looked to their source. They realized that their health did not originate with a drug program and none was needed to restore it!

A-I-D-S OR X-Y-Z?

At one point in the writing of this book, the authors considered this title:

THEY CONQUERED
AIDS/ARC,
HIV &
XYZ!

What does this mean?

The Persons who conquered these dread diseases—our "Conquerors"—achieved this much-desired goal with:
A PASSION FOR LIFE — SPIRITUAL ENLIGHTEN-MENT—and NATURAL THERAPIES—all a part of Holistic Healing.

These paths and methods are applicable to every other physical and mental disease and problem of mankind!

That is one meaning of "XYZ." It means "Etc."

***** "XYZ" *****

The victors over AIDS/ARC who tell their life stories practiced holistic healing. Their physical condition was accelerating toward death. But they recovered with this New Age form of healing that TREATS THE WHOLE PERSON—not only the body (with natural methods), but also the mind and the spirit.

The prevention of disease is an important part of holistic health. Practicing these principles can keep one well. Indeed, the ultimate goal in health is preventing disease, not attempting to cure it.

***** "XYZ" *****

Given a laboratory diagnosis of AIDS, some persons immediately commit suicide. The acronym AIDS alone triggers this terror of a disease considered to be invariably fatal. The common concept of AIDS is one of horrible suffering and a prolonged, painful death. The suicides prefer immediate death.

The acronym "AIDS", its predecessor HTLV-III, and other acronyms the virologists may yet come up with, might as well be "XYZ." The acronym "AIDS" has an assumed power through widespread publicity.

Not in the medical world, but in the world of holistic healing, AIDS is being proven to be not a death sentence, but an opportunity for greater growth and a higher level of consciousness. Repeatedly our "Conquerors" have confirmed this fact.

There exists an epidemic of extreme, unreasonable fear, a mesmerism of suggestion. This acronym "AIDS" has evolved into a synonym for fear of the unknown, helplessness before a universal, omnipotent contagion, and certain death. Also, there is a sense of an invisible, indestructible virus, or many viruses, replicating themselves, attacking the interior of the body, advancing armies slowly consuming their host.

If we could change the name of the disease "AIDS" to "XYZ," would much of its power disappear?

***** "XYZ" *****

It is not logical to believe that a healthy person can "catch" AIDS and in three months be dead. But this has happened. In such cases, is it the mesmerism of fear or is it the medical treatment—or both—that causes the death?

"XYZ" doesn't have any meaning, as we know it. It does not connote condemnation by the self or society, fear of the unknown, hopelessness, or certain death. But all of these are included in the acronym "AIDS."

***** "XYZ" *****

We are told that AIDS is a disease based on "signs and symptoms" and laboratory verification. There are many components to this disease that differ from other diseases. AIDS is called a disease, but it is actually a combination of diseases, so consequently the symptom picture is seldom the same. A person who dies with a diagnosis of AIDS might well die of the following: Kaposi's sarcoma (cancer), *pneumocystis carinii* pneumonia (PCP), a protozoan infection in the lungs, formerly rare; a rampant infection throughout the body due to a suppressed immune system; organ malfunction, due to disease processes; uremia or other poisoning; dementia.

The symptom picture for diagnosing AIDS is not clearly defined. There is much conjecture as to diagnosis and the "signs and symptoms."

Just before death, the heart stops pumping and/or the patient stops breathing. The true fact is that people are not dying of AIDS, but of either cardiac arrest or respiratory arrest!

The Merck Manual, principal guide to diagnosis, signs, symptoms and treatment for the medical profession, is updated constantly. But in the latest edition, the large section on the immune system is full of conjecture and theory.

Dr. Scott Gregory has counseled patients who are so fear-ridden by the picture presented in the media and by the medical profession, that they ask: "Why am I not experiencing the symptoms that are supposed to invariably accompany AIDS?" But soon they do manifest the symptoms through the power of their imagination! (See pages 313-314.)

Some individuals who are diagnosed as being HIV-Positive have more severe symptoms than those who have been diagnosed as having Kaposi's sarcoma. Some persons with "K.S." (purple lesions on the skin) have no other symptoms, and feel well. The conclusion is that AIDS in itself is complicated, we still have much to learn, and no one has the complete answer as to what is actually going on, and how different people react.

Therefore, no doctor should give absolutes to patients, such as: "You have six months to live." One patient of Dr. Gregory was told this by a prominent AIDS specialist at UCLA. But there is no time limit on life for certain, and doctors should not "play God."

In the book *Love, Medicine & Miracles*,[1] Dr. Bernie Siegel writes an open letter from patients to physicians. He says: "I

---

[1] Siegel, M.D., Bernie S. *Love, Medicine & Miracles,* page 127. (See Bibliography.)

advise patients to insist on (this) Patients' Bill of Rights." The letter starts: "Dear Doctor," and includes these lines: "Do not tell me how long I have to live! I alone can decide how long I will live."

Symptoms and Causes

"For every thousand persons hacking at the leaves of evil— there is only one person hacking at the roots."

—Henry David Thoreau

This truth applies to health and disease. When we treat symptoms, we are "hacking at the leaves of (disease.)" To "hack at the roots" is to remove the causes of the disease, by looking at the lifestyle of the patient and advising him to correct it, so that health returns naturally, and is maintained through wise and wholesome living.

On Drugs

"I firmly believe that if most of the pharmacopaeia were sunk to the bottom of the sea, it would be all the better for Mankind and all the worse for the fishes."

—Oliver Wendell Holmes, famous physician.

"Doctors pour drugs of which they know little—to cure diseases of which they know less—into human beings of whom they know nothing."

—Francois de Voltaire

"The doctor of the future will give no medicine, but will interest his patients in the care of the human body, in diet, and in the cause and prevention of disease."
—Thomas Alva Edison

"Physicians of the utmost fame
Were called at once, but when they came
They answered, as they took their fees,
'There is no cure for this disease'."

—Hilaire Belloc (1870-1953)

The Motives and Methods of Medical Doctors

We believe that the majority of medical doctors are motivated by a selfless love of humanity and a dedication to their profession. However, they are largely <u>mistaught</u>, from the years of medical school onward, as to the origins of disease and the best treatments for it. We do not impugn their MOTIVES, but many of their METHODS. Some enlightened medical doctors are now saying that it is the <u>system</u> that is at fault—a <u>medical monolith</u> has developed of such proportions that all—doctors and patients alike—are its victims.

Inspiring, true life stories follow—in the Conquerors' own words. Here are cases where Persons With AIDS discovered something completely new to them—the world of Holistic Healing.

It is hoped the stories of these "Conquerors" will serve as a pilot to help others find their way to restored health from a new basis—NATURAL AND SPIRITUAL THERAPIES.

Louie Paul Nassaney

Louie Paul Nassaney personifies the idea:

FROM SELF-RELIANCE—THRU INSPIRATION
—INTO TRANSFORMATION

Louie had reached a precipice between life and death in his struggle with the dread disease AIDS.

He abandoned reliance upon the medical regime that gave him no hope of recovery, but whose drugs had sent his body into a decline toward death.

He developed SELF-reliance. He found inspiration in his religion, new strength in exercise and sports, and mentors in the Holistic Health movement who showed him new paths and healing modalities. He was victorious over the disease.

His driving motivations are totally healing himself and helping others to discover more health and life.

Louie has a passion to live, free of disease; a passion to live on a higher level; a passion to share his hard-won knowledge with others, especially Persons with AIDS.

He is a spokesman for the survivors—Persons Who Have Conquered AIDS.

Louie Paul Nassaney's Adventure

There was a time—and it wasn't very long ago—when I thought I had everything. I was a member of a close-knit, loving family. I have a mom and dad, two brothers and two sisters. I worked in our family business, and it gave me an excellent income. A beautiful home, a fabulous car, fine clothes, friends, an active social life, lots of recreational drugs—all were mine. I had everything the media tell us to want—the things that are supposed to bring fulfillment and joy. How could it be, then, that I was not happy?

I had never told my family that I was gay, but I indulged in relationship after relationship, and between them, I played around. I suppose, according to some people's standards I was promiscuous, but I didn't think so at the time. My sex life was the norm according to my lifestyle. I believed I had many friends; they and I all lived the same way. If a relationship didn't satisfy me, I simply moved on to the next man. I didn't think about my affairs more than superficially. It was all part of being gay; I was merely doing what everyone else was doing and I didn't see it as a problem. After all, didn't I have everything? I never thought seriously about my own opinion of myself. It wasn't an issue. More important was what kind of impression I made on others, and that impression became my opinion of myself.

It was inevitable as I grew older: I realized that the imprint gays made on society was negative. Then I began to question my own standards. My self-imposed secrecy as to my lifestyle fostered a lack of self-love. The guilt, blame and shame grew daily subliminally; I never gave it a conscious thought. At the time I believed I was healthy, and yet I was abusing my body with a junk food diet. My parents ate the same way, so I was the second generation on this deficient, harmful diet. I was as careless about my health as I was about my feelings and the feelings of others. I believe this lifestyle contributed to a weakened immune system and was, in part, the reason that I eventually succumbed to AIDS.

In May of 1983, Dr. John Medved, in private practice in Santa Monica, diagnosed me as having Kaposi's sarcoma and AIDS. Dr. Medved sent me to UCLA and I was seen by Dr. Ron Mitsuyasu. The blood tests showed a lowered immune system. The doctors saw a spot, and did a biopsy on it. It was definite, there was no mistake...I had AIDS.

I turned to my family. The same day I was diagnosed I told my folks: "I am gay, and I have AIDS." Each member of my family in turn expressed his or her love for me and a desire to support me in all ways. My family has been my best support throughout this crisis. This disease has brought us even closer and my confidence in my family is total. I believe I am most fortunate to have a family willing to accept me and love me unconditionally. The love my family gave me helped me to learn to love myself, and that is the beginning of healing. Throughout this entire experience, my family supported me in every way. I moved in with them. I didn't have to worry about money.

Dr. Mitsuyasu arranged for me to receive the traditional treatment for AIDS. I was given a choice of chemotherapy or the drug Interferon.

I was encouraged to take part in a government program. Its purpose was to test the effects of the new drug Interferon on AIDS. I was told the drug was very expensive but I could get it free on this program. I thought if I didn't participate, I would definitely die, and soon. I was told the drug might save my life and that it was the only hope left to me. So gratefully, I agreed to allow the doctors to experiment on me with Interferon.

There was no reference to diet—and I was not given counseling for the terrible emotional stress I endured. I suffered from depression, anger, and fear. I had nightmares. I thought I was dying, and no positive thoughts concerning life came to my mind. For seven months I was hospitalized under the Interferon treatment. I was bedridden, unable to move about. My vision became blurred and got steadily worse. I couldn't hear well. My sense of touch was numbed. I lost my sense of taste and almost lost my sense of smell. I experienced a loss of coordination and found even walking extremely difficult. My hair fell out. I was taking sixteen to twenty-four Tylenol tablets a day and sleeping twelve to fifteen hours a day. I admit I had thoughts of suicide to avoid the pain and suffering, but I am a Roman Catholic, so suicide was really out of the question for me. My waking moments were spent in pain, fear, anger, and total depression. I was completely demoralized.

After seven months of hospital treatment, the doctors decided to take me off the drug Interferon. It wasn't working for me. I thought it was the only hope, and when it didn't work, I believed all hope was lost, that a death sentence had been issued.

The medical doctors advised me to start chemotherapy and radiation and said that possibly other experimental drugs might be helpful. But, they added, the prognosis was not good. It was at this point that I took control of my body. I decided that I didn't want to die full of drugs, chemicals and radiation. If I were going to die, let my death be natural. I told the doctors I would not submit to the treatment they advised. It was January, 1984, and I have not returned to any of those treatments, to any hospital or drugs.

As with most people facing death, my religion became very important to me. I attended mass daily and was in constant prayer. I guess I hadn't really given up on myself, because I prayed daily for guidance on how to live each day and find a path to health. My religion has been a source of great comfort and peace. I am grateful.

I was amazed to find that within the first month of freedom from the drug Interferon, I began to feel somewhat better. It was during the second month of freedom from the drug that my body began to wake up. About that time, a friend offered to give me a body massage. He was a very good friend to be willing to massage the body of a person with AIDS. More than that, while he massaged my body, he began to talk to me about letting go of the toxins within. He told me that the seven months I had been in the hospital the toxins had been sitting along my bones and arteries, so to speak. He spoke of meditation and relaxation, positive imagery and the healing of the spirit. I have always been a positive person, and as I heard these things, I began to learn to live one day at a time. I began to be grateful for each day of life I was being given. Positive information was beginning to come to me. Someone brought me a flyer from Louise Hay about her book *AIDS: A Positive Approach* . It was the first time I had heard that I could get well. It was all I needed to hear.

Louise Hay teaches meditation, relaxation, and healing imagery. She also emphasizes the need for a correct diet. I found a good nutritionist and began to get my diet on the right track. For the first time in my life, I began to eat correctly. I became very conscious of nutrition as a source of health. I believe it was a reflection of my self-love that I began to care, finally, about how I treated my body. The days of alcohol, cocaine, marijuana, and quaaludes were over forever. Instead of yielding to death, I began to explore the possibility of life. Each new understanding opened another door. I discovered the benefits of vitamin therapy, acupuncture, colonics, carrot juice, garlic and fasting. I focused on methods of stimulating my immune system.

The healing didn't happen all at once. I found I had to seek out the sources of health and become my own doctor.

Louise Hay emphasizes the absolute need to rid one's life of all negative stress, which creates illness. If we are to regain our health it is absolutely necessary to rid our lives of such stress. But how could I live with a supposedly terminal illness and not have stress in my life? That seemed impossible. I took the approach that I would live each day given to me to the fullest. Yes, there were times when I couldn't sustain the positive attitude; I suffered fear and depression, and the nightmares returned. I worked on emphasizing the positives and working through the negatives by anticipating days of joy and pleasure and the renewed health coming to me.

It was during this time that I found it necessary to free myself from all relationships not supportive and positive. My old friends had reacted predictably to my illness. They were frightened. They had dropped me like a stone, so I did the same with them. I began to surround myself with positive and supportive people who understood my constant efforts to improve my health. To be with positive-thinking people is now absolutely essential to my life. The lifestyle of my "old" friends would have killed me, and I would not die for their sakes.

I began to change—mentally, emotionally, and spiritually. I started on the journey to true self-love. Mentally, I try to keep my thoughts under control; I express love and kindness to others as well as to myself.

Physically, I began to do all I could to stimulate my immune system. I worked out at a gym. I took up body building, aerobics, racquetball and swimming. Then I added body surfing and bicycling. When you physically stimulate the immune system, it produces a corresponding mental and spiritual awakening and the endorphins within become activated. Physical exercise for me was essential.

I work hard at loving people. I refuse to indulge in thoughts of criticism, fear, anger, blame, shame, and guilt. I let people know that if they have such thoughts and emotions, they can choose another way to think and feel. It's not wrong to have negative thoughts, but it is wrong to get stuck in them. It is necessary to work through negative thinking in order to become free from it. People can choose love, joy, pleasure, and health. Both the negative and the positive always exist. It is our individual decision which to choose for our lives. This applies to everyone, not only to people who are facing death. A positive attitude is the foundation of healing spiritually, physically, and mentally.

People hear the word "healing" and they expect to see the lesions or other manifestations disappear immediately. But that isn't the point. It is not the right goal. A higher quality of life on every level is to be desired—not just saving our lives in order to continue to live destructively. On any particular day, if you feel good, take advantage of it. Give thanks, exercise, see loving friends, exult in the good days in every way you know. People with a death-expectant attitude, people who are unwilling to change their lifestyles, or make any effort—cannot be victorious over AIDS. People who succumb to the threat of death like to say they are "going to die with dignity." I say live with dignity. Life is for the living.

As to the disease itself: in my case it was sexually transmitted. I believe my immune system was weak to begin with. My lifestyle, eating habits, and mental attitude all contributed to a low level of health. I believed I was a healthy person then, but now I know that my immune system was being weakened in many ways. My uncaring, unfeeling, unknowing lifestyle was one of them.

At the age of twenty-one, I acquired sexually transmitted hepatitis. I was not given any drugs, but merely told to go home and rest. I don't think I took the illness seriously and did not take time to see it totally healed. I spent two weeks in bed and then returned to my former lifestyle which included cocaine, quaaludes, some marijuana and alcohol. I believe my lifestyle and mental attitude contributed to the disease of AIDS.

I don't believe that AIDS is a "gay" disease. I believe it

has gone through the gay community, but is not limited to nor did it originate in the gay community.

I have heard the rumor that the virus was introduced into society intentionally, directed toward those people the U.S. society feels the most hostility towards—the gay community and the non-white community. I certainly hope it isn't true. It could be true, but that is the kind of rumor I refuse to dwell on.

Each of us is an individual, mentally, spiritually, and physically. Because the medical community refuses to consider any modality other than drug therapy to heal AIDS, it is necessary for each of us to take control of his own body and seek the methods that work for us. There are those who respond to radiation, chemotherapy, and drugs. I did not. But you may. Realize that if what you are doing isn't working for you, there are many, many other things you can do to help yourself.

But it won't be handed to you. You have to get out there and find out what will work for you. It is essential that you become absolutely honest with yourself. You must consider seriously how far you are willing to go to regain your health. As for me, I will go all the way. I found in myself a strength where I was 100% willing to take whatever steps were necessary to live even one more day.

I was and am willing to change myself and my lifestyle in whatever way good health requires. This means getting rid of the poisons in my life—mental, physical, and emotional poisons. It means a change in priorities—a total change in diet and daily activities. I am willing and I will try—for the sake of living another day. Being willing to do that, gives me a chance to live. That was and is my attitude toward myself.

I believe that there is no help for those with a poor attitude. You must believe in what you are doing—believe that it will work. That belief is of the utmost importance. Every day, every hour, every minute of my life I am reaching for a quality of life that I did not know existed before AIDS. Quality, not quantity, is the name of this game. The most important thing I could say to a person with AIDS is: if you feel good in the morning, get out there and take advantage of it. Be grateful and live completely today. Stimulate your life, and you will stimulate your mind, body, and your immune system.

When we are young, we usually do not consider dying. Those thoughts are for the old ones whose lives have been lived, and they are ready. When a young person is surprised by the possibility of an early death—when tomorrow becomes a dream—today takes on another dimension.

Wouldn't it be wonderful if everyone on this planet could find out what many people with AIDS have been forced to learn? Why do we have to face death before we learn about the value of life? We must learn to live truly in the moment. We must learn to live for each minute, hour, and day with gratitude and take full advantage of every good feeling and good time the world has to offer. We should wake up each morning grateful for another day, and if we feel good, run to take advantage of all the joys of life. Hurry up and learn to give love and be kind to others and seek the God within us all. I have learned to be grateful for the gift of this disease. Each day I live I feel like a "winner." I have truly found a great joy in life. This disease has been a gift of life to me. I know that some people find that difficult to believe—but it is true, nevertheless. I have found a new awareness, and how to live on higher levels, with love, joy, and expectancy.

In one month, several friends died of AIDS. I became depressed in my grief. I began to slack off on my diet, and stopped going to the gym to work out. I allowed my thinking to go negative. My whole regimen began to slip, and the disease attacked me again. The symptoms began to return. I had to get hold of myself quickly and return to my health-generating activities. I did so, and the disease retreated. I know now that it will be necessary for me to live all my days doing battle against this disease in the sense that I cannot ever return to my former lifestyle. I cannot ever allow depression, fear, blame, shame, and guilt to seep into my heart, mind, and body. I must be ever alert and on guard.

A great thinker has written, "Stand porter at the door of thought." I am willing to do all I can to support life and I will not willingly succumb again to the negative thoughts and actions that will indeed kill me. If I don't eat properly and think properly and constantly do all that I can to stimulate my immune system, I will be vulnerable to attack. I am not talking about a cure—I am talking about a new lifestyle.

I hope this disease will cause a change in the medical world's approach to healing. Dr. Bernie Siegel's book, *Love, Medicine & Miracles* is a beginning. It shows there are some medical doctors who are beginning to see the light. It seems obvious that drugs do not heal everything. A new method for coping must be developed. It is necessary to take a more complete look at the art of healing and our concepts of man. The body is matter, that's true—but we are not just bodies—we are also mental, emotional and spiritual beings.

Wouldn't it be intelligent of the medical community to take a wider look at healing and include in its art the methods now considered "alternative?" At this point it is necessary for persons with AIDS to doctor themselves. The medical world has closed its mind to anything other than drugs. Yet, the natural, "alternative" methods are very old—and it seems to me that if a method is very old—it has lasted because IT WORKS!

Must the medical world be faced with a plague before it can change its beliefs regarding the various ways to heal? Must a human being be confronted with death before he/she can open the mind to a change in lifestyle?

Healing the spirit is the beginning of healing the body. Right thinking can bring about healing.

How can one's health not be affected by diet? How long must we wait, and how many of us will suffer and die before a crack is made in the monolithic establishment—with its current practices of drugs, radiation, and chemotherapy? The responsibility falls on each one of us.

We are in the forefront of this change in healing practices. The burden of responsibility lies with each of us—infected individuals or the healthy. We must seek out true healing and insist that it be practiced in all its aspects. AIDS could have a positive effect on the world if the medical complex would open its doors to other healing methods and use drugs only where they really work—in emergency situations to save lives.

Because of my changes in thinking, feeling, and acting, I have discovered I am able to make a total commitment. I have been in a personal relationship for some time. We are totally honest with each other; my lover is familiar with all aspects of my illness. We practice "safe sex." Yet I don't really know what "safe" sex is. I don't honestly believe condoms are safe. I'm told they are ninety percent safe, but there is that questionable ten percent. We just don't know. For myself, I take any and all precautions to protect my lover. We enjoy sex, but sex is not the foundation of our relationship—friendship is.

I keep myself active and feel well and strong. But I know that I must be extremely careful. Because I had cancer (K.S. is a form of cancer), I must watch my diet, live an unstressed life, and carry on my entire lifestyle in a way that is not disease-inducing but is health promoting. I feel healthy, but some K.S. lesions remain (as of May, 1988).

As to my future—I am writing a book, and books as you know, can take years to complete. I refuse to give any urgency or stress to this project, however, and will take my time to do it right. But the book isn't my only project. I no longer work from eight to five. I spend time learning about this disease and also developing myself spiritually.

The most fulfilling thing for me is to be able to help others—especially Persons With AIDS—with what I have learned. I have always enjoyed teaching and lecturing—helping to open doors to the possibilities of life for another person.

There are only a few leaders in the gay community who are able to speak from experience concerning this killing disease. The number will no doubt grow, but in the meantime, I have the feeling this is my path. I feel responsible to my fellows to get as much information as I can to those who still suffer. It is a very rewarding way of life.

Today is all I have and I intend to make the most of it. Tomorrow is still a dream, and it will take care of itself.

*   *   *   *   *

Note: Louie Nassaney appeared on The Oprah Winfrey Show, April 5, 1988, and gave his story. He also was featured in "Surviving Is What I Do", in *Time* magazine, May 2, 1988.

WHAT LOUIE NASSANEY DID

• He found out how healing actually occurs, on all levels: physical, mental, emotional and spiritual.

• After a near-death experience with immuno-suppressive therapies and drugs, he rejected them.

• He learned that a positive attitude is the foundation of healing oneself; he practiced and proved it.

• He learned about health and how to maintain it. He is in excellent health today.

• He started loving himself. (His family had always loved and accepted him unconditionally, and that helped him to learn to love himself.)

• He developed a nourishing sexual, sensual relationship but found it doesn't always have to end in coitus.

• He maintained a healthful diet and learned how to do this with correct foods and supplements.

• He stopped all toxic input: tobacco, caffeine, sugar, salt, alcohol, drugs, all medication. He avoided negative people and negative emotions which include criticism, anger, guilt, hopelessness, and despair.

• He improved his mind by learning and working with inner strengths.

• He nourished his heart by enhancing personal, loving relationships.

• He improved his spiritual orientation by finding factors such as inspiring people, books, groups, and lifestyles.

• He improved all activity levels: aerobics (oxygenating the body), relaxation, physical exercise, sports. He learned that physical exercise is essential to stimulate the immune system.

• He learned about holistic healing and how to use natural modalities.

• He believed in what he was doing, believed that it would work.

• Louie Paul Nassaney experienced a rebirth—physical, emotional, and spiritual.

Russell John Carlton

The first thing you notice when you see Russell John Carlton is his eyes. They burn with an intensity that speaks of a deep involvement with life, a need for it and a dedication to it. Then you become aware that here before you is a strapping young man of 25 years filled with terrific energy and vitality. Six feet tall with not an excess pound on his body, he seems the epitome of health. Yet his life has been filled with sorrows, bizarre happenings, uncertainties, pain, and disease. How did he overcome the problems that touched him in his early school years? He was robbed for a time of the love of his parents when he was a sensitive youth.

What strengths did he find that now he stands so confident? How did he learn to face his gayness and accept himself? Sometimes it takes great sorrow to lift us to the life we were meant to live.

Russell John Carlton's Adventure

Being gay in this day and age, even though it seems more accepted, is still very hard, because not only do we have to deal with non-acceptance from our peers, from the society we live in, from our families, but also, from ourselves. Many people do not come to terms with the truth about themselves, whatever it may be. It's hard to be openly gay, but to keep hiding your lifestyle is a stressful way to live. This stress in my life later manifested in poor health.

When I was very young, like most children, I had no problems. Life was beautiful, and so was the world I lived in. I loved my parents very much, and they loved me. My home was warm and filled with happiness. When did it change? I can't really say; I only know it changed.

My early school life was unhappy. I was a sickly kid, scrawny and sensitive. I passed from one grade to another until finally I reached high school. I went to school in Scottsdale, Arizona. The kids, for the most part, came from wealthy homes and made sure that you fit into their society or you were mocked. I became heavily involved with theatre and the yearbook—in fact, with all the arts the school had to offer. I wasn't the jock type. I was sensitive, and soon was tagged with the name "faggot" or "gay" or whatever. I'm not effeminate, but when I was in high school, I was still on the scrawny side, and the name stuck. Young people can be very cruel, sometimes without even realizing it, but often it's deliberate. In my case, throughout high school, I was picked on a lot and some really bizarre things happened. I was sexually molested by an older man when I was only sixteen. I had emotional hangups from this for some time. The act in itself was bad enough but he was traveling with the theater group I was with. He forced himself on me, and he was a married man. It really shook me up quite a bit.

I was young, but I realized I had to get some answers if

I was going to survive. I knew all my life that I was gay, but I still refused to face it until one day I said to myself, "Listen, there's a God, and He loves me the way I am—and if I'm this way, how can it be so wrong?" I had had it with judgments from my peers. Some of the ones I hung around with turned out to be gay themselves. In high school, if you're different, or veer from the norm, kids will exaggerate your differences, and make your life miserable. My high school life was therefore not the happiest. When I finally left high school, I wanted to get as far away from those people as I could.

I was facing my gayness at this point in my own consciousness, but I had not declared it openly. The world I lived in seemed to "accuse" me of it, but I had made no commitment. One day I said to myself, "Come on, let's face it, I'm gay, and I want to get on with my life." I was eighteen years old when I finally told my parents. They loved me very much, and I knew they loved me, but they were unable to deal with it. I felt hurt, rejected and terribly depressed. It may have been my lover who caused their lack of acceptance. They may have understood what I didn't—that it was a destructive relationship and, consequently, they held him responsible for the turn my life had taken.

My depression continued. I really was confused about love, about my lover and me, and about life. My lover seemed to be jealous of my artistic ability and convinced me that I would be better off to give up art, which I did. This only added to my confusion and depression, I'm sure. All my life I had been artistic and expressed myself in the arts; now I was being robbed of them by my lover. Yet, I was in collusion with the robber, for I had robbed myself, although I did not realize it at the time. I needed love as we all do. Perhaps I tried to substitute the feeling my lover had for me for the lost love of my parents. I was grasping at anything that would put purpose in my life. There was nothing to grasp, nothing to hold on to. My parents were gone; my art was gone, and my dreams—I had no dreams any more. I just didn't care. I kept giving up. I didn't want to live.

My depressions increased; I lost weight. I have somehow felt that I was stricken with AIDS because I created it out of depression, a lack of self-love, lack of purpose, and, in short, because my life was just a void. I felt no hope, and I looked forward to no future. So I created my illness.

I had three doctors: a surgeon, an internist, and a family physician. I would go to one of them, and he would give me tests. Then another would want to see me, and there were more tests. They were worried. They thought I was becoming precancerous. They thought I had Hodgkin's disease. I remained depressed. The relationship with my lover was not a good one, but I was too down to realize it or care. My thoughts were suicidal when I became ill, so I let the condition overtake me even more. I just didn't want to live. I wanted disease to overcome me. I didn't rail against fate, or blame anyone for my condition. I was in a self-destructive mode.

This is a difficult situation for medical doctors to handle. I developed more adverse symptoms. I had mononucleosis for six months. It became chronic. My doctor told me I had to give up my job, or I would become very, very sick. I did leave that job, and my symptoms lessened. I took another job, and six months later, I relapsed into a whole new set of symptoms. I developed adenopathy from the mononucleosis. My blood levels, my lymphocytes, were down. The minerals in my blood were very low. My adenopathy developed into tumors. The swelling in my lymph nodes stayed, and stubbornly refused to go away. I had severe weight loss. I'm just under six feet. When I was my sickest, I weighed only 122 pounds. I was very thin. I had dizzy spells and blackouts in addition to gastritis and diarrhea. I was jaundiced and bilious. I was just melting away.

My doctors didn't seem to know what was wrong with me. They had come to a mutual conclusion that something was definitely wrong, but they didn't have the answers. They linked me with some rare lymphoma which they thought I had contracted from a cat. They said my lymphatic system was chronically damaged. As I mentioned, I did have tumors and adenopathy. The doctors did a biopsy. They removed a tumor from my groin, which proved to be benign. They did a complete series of tests and all my blood work. I was going from one thing to another, and they couldn't tell me what was wrong with me. All they could do was pump me full of drugs and take my money. I was becoming even more depressed. A sickness like that works on your mind, too.

All the things that were happening in my life seemed to erode my self-esteem. I felt I was the one to blame, only myself. I was always the one. When things went wrong, filling me with frustrations and inharmonies, I always accused myself: "It's me. It's me!" I'd say. In addition, I felt like a social outcast. I would think, "Who wants to be around me? I have this disease." I call this period of my life my "dark ages."

Surely, my spirit was dead. I think a big part of AIDS deals with the spiritual side of each one of us. AIDS strikes each one of us differently. I've seen some people die in a week. Some people have hung on for a year, and some have hung on for four or five years, and then turned the odds around. I think AIDS stems from a lack of self-love, as any disease does, because if you truly believe in the power of love, and you emanate that love, there is no room for disease. I feel strongly about this because of my own experience. Yes, if your body, mind, and spirit are receptive, that is, out of balance, and the opportunity is right, AIDS will take you and take you fast!

But I was lucky. I was young, and the disease was young. In 1981, medical doctors were not using the term AIDS when diagnosing. It was a new disease; they didn't know what it was. The name hadn't been decided on, so my doctor did not call it AIDS. But later, doctors said, due to my signs and symptoms, it no doubt had been AIDS. About this time in searching for an alternative method, I encountered holistic medicine. My medical doctors wanted to perform more tests, and presumably, some operations. I couldn't stand the thought of them cutting me up any more, so I refused.

I was so weak when I was released from the County General Hospital, there was nothing I could do. I was so weak that my lover had to help me walk to the car. But I decided I wanted it—I wanted to live. At the beginning, I felt I was going to die, but now I wanted to live. It was a whole new turn-around.

AIDS is a very dark disease. It's catastrophic in the way it attacks. It moves in and overcomes you. The society we live in today, with drug abuse, sexual promiscuity, and excesses of all kinds is unbalanced, making us open to disease. I think the reason AIDS took such a strong hold on the gay community is because the gay lifestyle, even in this day and age, is very hard. Many gays do not come to terms with themselves. This is stressful. That's why I believe night life is so common on the gay side. And incidentally, why AIDS was originally linked only with the gay lifestyle. Night life is the one way a gay person can lift the "bricks" off his shoulders. He can be free. He's with his own kind. He can relax, drink, etc., and not bother about being censored. I really think that's one of the reasons there's so much sexual activity. It's an expression of freedom, a freedom that gay people want and can experience. Gay men have many sexual partners. Once, it was something to be proud of—the many sexual partners and activities one engaged in. It was something very socially accepted. In fact, if you didn't follow this example, you were almost looked down upon.

So when it first appeared, AIDS was considered a disease that struck only the homosexual. Of course, that is not true. The situation made the homosexual more susceptible. Stress alone can be a killing thing; I feel that it was the stress involved in being gay that was the killer. I feel that anyone who is living a life of stress is laying himself wide open to illness. I believe that AIDS touches everyone in some way. But the public tried to confine it to a specific group of people. It is like that all through history. Some people are always persecuted; it doesn't matter who you are or what you are. Disease does not restrict itself to any one group.

Heart disease, stress, cancer—these are at all time highs. They strike anywhere. We live at such a fast pace, and bombard our bodies with junk foods. We're a nation of wealth—but much sickness.

We abuse our bodies with the air we breathe, with the nicotine, alcohol, and drugs we take into our bodies. It's a miracle that we exist at all. I'm not judging, believe me. I've been there. I was never promiscuous sexually, but I dabbled in drugs. I think the biggest thing I ever did was a little speed. I did cocaine a few times, and a little marijuana, but it was minimal. When I was in high school, I never touched it at all, any of it. After I moved out to Los Angeles, I experimented more, but it's been very moderate, because I know about drugs and what they can do. Still, I was under stress and like the rest of the civilized world, and especially the gay world because the need was greater, I was searching for meaning and freedom.

If this seems like a digression, it isn't really, because these were the thoughts that occupied my mind when I was being treated by orthodox medicine. My condition worsened daily, and I was reaching out for an alternate method. Then I found the holistic methods and had to learn to adapt them to my problems. Something new always holds the shadow of the unknown. You rationalize. You try to think your way out of a situation you find yourself in. That's what I was doing. Holistic medicine finally became the answer—because every way I looked at it, everywhere I turned my thoughts, it made sense. We are not just physical bodies. Our body has needs, our mind has needs, and our spiritual self also has needs. Treating only one of these aspects, I came to realize, doesn't make sense.

Among the doctors who helped me in the holistic

method was my chiropractor. He was one person of prime importance. He opened doors for me. His responsibility was to open doors; my responsibility was to walk through them. Many doors can be opened for people, but if they don't walk through them, they can't experience what's on the other side. This doctor laid the tools in front of me in such a way that I decided to pick them up and use them. That's the main factor with support that people don't realize. The patient must be involved, must contribute, must pick up the tools.

I firmly believe that was when I started to get well. I was suddenly getting wonderful support from my chiropractor, my nutritionist, my iridologist, my colon therapist, my new lover, and many others. When I got rid of my destructive relationship, my parents welcomed me back. This was and still is very important to me. We love each other very much. Now they are supportive of me. It took time, but we are now close again. They have met my lover and like him. These may seem like small things, but they are all part of a happy life, a good way of life. My depressions left me. I was preparing a better battleground for my struggle to overcome AIDS. I had not won the war against AIDS, but I had won one battle. I wanted to live!

The group of holistic doctors I was involved with were very supportive and thorough. I had a curvature in my spine which was possibly causing problems with my pancreas. I was anemic along with everything else. They linked it all together. I learned a lot.

One of the first things I did was to go on a carrot juice fast with distilled water and herbs—for six days. It was the most tremendous week. The fast arrested my fever. It was a hard thing for me to stay on, but I went through it. During the fasting, I had colonics.

Then I went on a rigorous diet program. I wasn't able to eat protein. So instead of cow's milk I prepared and drank almond milk. I drank special herbal teas to heal my nervous, respiratory, and immune systems. The herbal teas were catnip, skullcap, red clover, chaparral and others. I didn't work; I didn't do anything else. I had lost my job because of my illness. I focused on recovering. I was able to really concentrate on myself, and all I wanted to do was to get well. Everything was upbeat. Everything was very encouraging.

One of the doctors told me of a woman who had a tumor the size of a grapefruit. The doctor said to her, "Listen, do you want to live?" She said she did. He put her on a fast and within a week she got her color back, and the tumor had started to reduce itself. It seems like a miracle, but it happens. I had tumors, and I dissolved them all. Even if someone feels he's going to die and is very discouraged, I believe fasting will arrest what's going on, because if you fast the process of autolysis goes on. You actually digest the disease. The first cells to go are your diseased cells. So I believe fasting is very, very powerful.[1]

Carrot juice is extremely valuable. I drink it to this day. It has enzymes; it is a living food.

I have heard that fasting has caused a number of deaths. Whether that statement has any truth or not, I don't know. Maybe they didn't understand fasting; maybe they didn't know what they were doing, and were unsupervised. Maybe, instead of a fast, they were following one of the current weird diets of the day.

I am convinced that a holistic way of life prevents and cures disease. A nutritious diet, including carrot juice, helps to insure a happy, progressive, and prolonged life.

I've never advised anyone to do anything, because I'm not a doctor. I give information from my life. I reach out to people who need help or comfort. I share my own experiences, my own positive thinking. In one of the national polls, it was found that many individuals who come down with disease feel

---

[1]See comments on fasting at end of chapter.

they're being punished in some way. I don't believe this. If the mind is not controlled, disease can take over. I try to help Persons With AIDS put thoughts like this out of their minds. Again, I think this disease stems from a lack of self-love. So many feel that, for whatever reason, they must punish themselves. If the mind, the body, and the spirit are in balance, it naturally follows that we do not judge or punish ourselves. I recommend that people read a positive, uplifting book along this line. I'll say, "Listen, you should read this. I think it will help you." But if they are interested in fasting or diet procedures, I always insist: "Check with your nutritionist." There are many weird diets. I don't believe in fasting to lose weight, especially without the advice of a doctor. I feel that many of these diets are unbalanced. Under supervision, on a juice diet, you're giving your body all it needs. The nutritionist explains to you that the week you fast, you have to take it easy. You're cleansing and healing yourself. Also, when you're on a fast, you drink lots and lots of water. I urinated all the time while fasting. You get headaches, you get nauseated, so you drink an enormous amount of water to keep flushing the poisons out. The disease will devour itself. Fasting gives it an opportunity to do so.

There is another factor in overcoming AIDS. If I hadn't had a complete turnaround, I might never have realized it. But, to repeat, holistic medicine is threefold. I know I was sick, not only in body but in mind and spirit as well. I believe the body is like a pyramid: your body, your mind, and your spirit, each forms a firm foundation for the other. If they're not working in unison, one will overbalance the others. The mind is very powerful, because we are creators. You create your own depression if you're not accepting who you really are. If you're not comfortable with yourself, then you are going to set up within yourself—in your consciousness—certain factors to make your life unbearable, and open to disease. I feel that in a sense I created my illness, because I gave it the conditions that nurtured it.

I abused myself through my lack of self-love. People need to learn a new awareness. They need to realize that, first of all, each of our bodies is a temple. We need to have our temples in order. We need to cultivate our mind, body, and spirit, making them one. People must realize that with this new knowledge, they can catapult themselves to a new level of awareness. They can learn to take care of themselves. First, love yourself and care for your body; then everything else falls into place. If you truly have an attitude of love, there is no room for disease.

That's what's so sad about "safe sex." The emotion behind sex is very important. Many people are basically still following the same self-indulgence and saying, "I'm going to be safe. I'm just going to put this rubber on, and I'll be safe." That's a bit ignorant because it's really not safe. There's an imbalance. There's a wrong thought behind "safe sex." I believe we need a new life approach about sex and what sex really means. Sex without love—I don't see how safe that can ever be. But sex with love, I think can be safe. I think it's the way people perceive sex, and where they operate from. Some go to the bathhouses, and think all they have to do is slip on a condom to practice "safe sex." I don't think that's the way it is. I think people are now regarding sex with a little more virtue, rather than mere sensation. They are realizing they must link love with sex. Sex as an expression of love can be very beautiful.

There are many aspects of disease, and especially of AIDS, because it encompasses many diseases. Some people who discover they have AIDS literally scare themselves to death. Their minds are overcome by fear, and they give in to that fear. They have AIDS; they are going to die. If I were going to advise them, I would say, "Don't give in to that panic or give it power." It's of the utmost importance, in my opinion, for people with AIDS to make peace with themselves, to decide what they want. Some people want to leave this earth. Some people want to fight; they want to live. I think each should make peace with his own belief, and not with anyone else's. Each should do what is right for himself. But I also believe people should look at other alternatives in viewing themselves. This comes from my own experience, of course. Most of all, I believe people should understand the power of love and accept the power they have, and not feel they have a fatal disease. The conviction that it is fatal will inevitably manifest itself in exactly that! The power of the mind! They can turn it all around to love and realize they can change it. People must accept and understand that this disease doesn't have them—they have it. It is just a temporary situation you can change. It isn't necessarily fatal. Don't close all the doors around you.

I believe that being human, we all have many basic responses: we can all smile, like the same song, feel the same emotions, and make choices. It may seem like a hard thing to say, but I think people's choices should be respected. I don't think it's a question of right or wrong. Some people think that AIDS is a karmic thing. They think it's time for them to go on, to come back later, perhaps with a better chance for happiness. Death is their choice. Others need a slap in the face to turn their life around. I was slapped, and I chose to live.

When I turned the sickness around, I turned my lifestyle around, and not just for the duration of the sickness. I have been totally well for about six years, and it's an on-going thing. When I was first sick in Arizona, holistic medicine wasn't as accepted as it is today. In seven years, holistic medicine has come a long way. I believe in it, and I continue to keep its precepts in my life. It brought me a whole new awareness about understanding, taking care of my body, and about life itself.

Sleep has become very important to me. What I eat is very important to me, but I try not to be obsessed with food. An obsession is an imbalance. It can become an enemy. I take supplements, minerals and vitamins. I'm trying to learn about food combining. I take herbs, and I'm constantly trying to do things to cleanse myself the best way I can.

There are certain things I will not eat: sugar[1], red meat[2], and most dairy products. I think sugar is really one of the nation's great health faults, and it's in almost everything. I understand that sugar erodes the immune system very quickly.

My bout with AIDS helped me in so many different ways. It changed my whole life, giving me a new strength, new courage, new direction, and a new power within myself. I learned about life, and what we can create. It even changed my physical appearance. At a fair, an old roommate of mine saw me. My lover and I had rented a place from him in Phoenix. I see him maybe once a year, because he comes to these festivals. He just can't believe I'm the same person, because physically, I've changed so much. I feel it's the inner change that is beginning to mold the outer. I can look in the mirror and love myself. I'm proud of who I am. That's all I can be, and I love myself. There are days when it's not as easy as other days, but I always remember I love myself. When you constantly judge and nag yourself, you're creating a snow-balling situation that can rob you of your life. Naturally, I go through the same trials and troubles as everybody else. I get a parking ticket, or something else happens to upset me, but it's always just a little upset, just for the moment. Formerly, I'd pick on myself 90 percent of the time, and ten percent of the time I loved myself. Now it's 90 percent I love myself, and ten percent, I don't, but that's part of being here. It's a lesson I still have to learn.

---

[1] See "The Truth About Sugar" at end of chapter.
[2] Volumes have been written about meat. Readers who would like information on nutrition, fasting, etc., write the Vegetarian Society, Inc., P.O. Box 126, Joshua Tree, CA 92252 — a non-profit organization. Please send $2.00 to cover costs.

I have become very steadfast in those things that are important for me. I need to learn about patience. Sometimes your mind thinks faster than you want it to. I've learned about the power of patience, of making it a friend instead of an enemy. The disease has changed my thinking. It's made me really watch others and try to share my experience with them, to let them know that if you have AIDS, you don't have to die! It's seriously made me realize much about power. We have much more power than we give ourselves credit for. I know now the things that really mean a great deal to me in life. This life offers such a variety of things and experiences. My lifestyle is to take care of myself in all areas. My sexual practices have changed, too. I was never promiscuous, and I've been in my current relationship about a year. It's monogamous. But I'm more cautious. I think twice. Sex with love is beautiful, and I place love above everything else, because love is God. Love is this earth, the flowers, a beautiful day. Love is the ocean, all nature. When you look at something beautiful, it gives you a sense of calming. Love is all-encompassing, and it's filled with peace. With love, I trust. Unconditional love is what it's all about. As each day goes by, I learn more.

The urgency has gone out of my life. I plan to continue living in Los Angeles for a while, and then I want to go somewhere a little more peaceful, a little more reclusive. I'm here for career purposes. When I feel the time is right, I'd like to move. But my living conditions must harmonize with my desire to enlighten myself continually. I live in Laurel Canyon in a peaceful environment. It's very quiet. There are trees and greenery, animals and birds. I love the bird songs I hear every day. I think it's necessary for people's health to have these natural things around them. Animals remind us where we've come from, and what life's really all about. I backpacked into the Grand Canyon to be able to look at nature just the way it is, to get fulfillment out of that. Man is always trying to change things and to manipulate the environment instead of just letting it be. If we could only realize what is there in nature—a healing force and power for us.

It's easy to be swept up into the turmoil of the crowd when you live in the city. The pace is fast; newspapers sell negative thoughts on every corner. I don't believe in poring over the newspapers. I try not to bombard myself with this kind of information, because most of it is very negative and depressing. I read it occasionally, but there are other things I feel are more important to read. The great and spiritual ideas are in books. I believe in my spiritual life. I believe in God. I also believe that if we were created in the image of God, we are God, too.

In my early years, I wanted to be an archeologist. Ancient and lost civilizations captured my imagination—collecting fossils, delving into the secrets of the ancient past. How old civilizations had lived, why they had disappeared, and what strange knowledge they had taken with them, were mysteries I wanted to solve. It was after this period of my life that I had a calling to the ministry. At one time, I wanted to become a Franciscan monk.

Perhaps it was my intrinsic leaning toward the religious that made me take to the holistic idea of curing the body and the mind. In my opinion, it was my mind that had created my illness, and my mind had to be healed. I do not mean to infer that my illness was not real. It definitely was. I can point to test after test that showed that illness. I merely want to stress the fact that healing became not only a physical, but a mental and spiritual matter also.

My spiritual conviction was the thing that saved me. I've always been religious. After I got well, I had a second calling to the ministry. But I realized again that this was not to be my path and that I could do it another way—with my art. When I was ill, this little voice inside wouldn't be stopped.

There were books on metaphysics I read that helped open more doors for me. One particular book called *The Nag*

Hammadi Library, an actual transcript of what Jesus wrote to his disciples, was very enlightening. It contains much the Bible leaves out. It's similar to *The Lost Books of the Bible*, *The Secret Life of Jesus*, *The Unknown Life of Jesus Christ* and *The Essene Gospel of Peace*. The "library" remains in the original form—before the Bible was rewritten. Religion puts God and Jesus in one place, and we're all here in another place. There's no way we can leave here until we die. But this book says that we are one with Jesus. He was an enlightened being. Because we are one with him, if we work at it, we can be where He is. I'm not saying it would be easy. I'm saying the potential is there, and it's worth striving for.

When you deal with the mind, the body and the spirit, you become aware of your great potentials. As this disease brought me closer to God, it brought me closer to my purpose in life and closer to some of the true virtues that I needed to express. It made me stronger in my philosophy and made me realize my potential in art. I learned about the power of creating my life and my surroundings. I found a new job, met new people, and was able to develop my career and my art work. I was much more secure within my knowledge of myself and my own identity, and was able to procure art assignments that showed me the importance of my art work. Perhaps because of my early religious leanings and my love of archeology and hidden things, my art uses metaphysics and symbology. I take symbols from the Egyptian, the Atlantean tradition, and astrology. I try to think of motifs from other philosophies and cultures, and integrate them into a contemporary symbology which tells stories pictorially, so there are no language barriers. People can look at my pictures and get a subliminal message. It's like transpersonal art. I use iridescent colors. People may not necessarily understand the message, but it gives them a nice, peaceful emotion inside. I want to share my creative art experience with the world. My lover and I have just finished painting a mural dedicated to the AIDS crisis. It's called "Blue Moon Trilogy." It's the human transformation that's occurring as a result of AIDS. The mural deals with it by declaring that together we can overcome any of our difficulties.

Everyone thought the AIDS situation was going to set us back 100 years, but I think it's going to project us forward 100 years, because people are really much more aware of what "gay" is. A good part of the arts and the wonderful things in life are provided by the sensitive people, and many of them are gay. This contribution is beginning to find appreciation in the world of New Thought.

WHAT RUSSELL JOHN CARLTON DID

• After a period of being extremely depressed and suicidal, he made a drastic turnaround in his consciousness, and decided that he wanted to live.

• He wasn't ready to leave this earth. He was young; he had work to do and a life to enjoy.

• He learned the power of true love.

• He learned the power of patience. Urgency has gone out of his life.

• He learned that disease is a temporary condition that can be changed.

• He learned that in reality, disease does not control the patient; he has control over it.

• He learned that the power of the mind is tremendous and largely unknown.

• After suffering from medical treatments, he rejected them in favor of natural therapies. These and a change in consciousness resulted in a holistic healing.

• He discovered the healing forces in nature.

• He realized that for a healing to take place, the entire being—body, mind, and spirit—must be addressed. The patient must become totally involved in his healing, and contribute to it.

• He stopped his destructive lifestyle—permanently.

• He dropped a destructive relationship, and found a new positive one.

• He found that sleep was important to him, for a complete sense of well-being.

• He took herbal supplements, vitamins and minerals and learned all he could about cleansing and detoxifying his body.

• After checking with a nutritional expert, he fasted from solid foods for six days. This period initiated his healing. The cleansing fast included carrot juice and special herbs.

• He eliminated sugar, red meat, and dairy products from his diet.

• What he learned about disease and health changed his entire life, giving him new strength, new courage, and new direction.

• He did not allow the negativity from the media to affect him. He read few newspapers and watched little television.

• His spiritual convictions helped to save him. He heard the "still, small voice" inside himself. This guided him.

• His spiritual growth helped him realize his potential in the arts. This desire to express himself helped him recover.

• He discovered his true identity.

• He reached out to others who needed help.

• He shared his own experiences and his own positive thinking.

• He believes that his disease partly stemmed from a lack of self-love.

• He realized that he had been abusive to himself—mentally and physically.

• He realized the power of the mind, and he took full responsibility for having created his illness.

• He learned a new awareness, that of accepting responsibility for the disease. (The corollary is that one can reverse disease.)

• Russell John Carlton developed a consciousness of true, spiritual love, and in that love, there is no room for disease.

*   *   *   *   *

Russell John Carlton is to be admired for his battle against a nearly fatal disease and for the solutions he chose to win that battle.

He shares further thoughts and inspirational messages with the reader here.

These writings give additional insight into how he overcame the dread disease. They show the thought quality of the transformation which occurred in his life, and which continues to shape it. So may the reader understand better this man, this healer of himself.

*   *   *   *   *

THE POWER IN AFFIRMATIONS

Now is the time to search your deepest thoughts, to finally see the unseen. Look into your heart and ask yourself what it is you truly want, what you feel is your purpose in this life. Take time, for every breath that you take and exhale, your thoughts will always follow.

Write down the affirmations you will make. Remember to cover everything, especially affirmations that deal with your illness. This is the tool you will use to help you surround yourself with the "White Healing Light" that you are going to need in this time of crisis.

Remember the space from whence you came... LOVE. You have the power within to heal yourself. Make your affirmations a daily prayer. Before you read them to yourself, relax, center your mind, then read them slowly aloud. Make your affirmations STRONG, for the words and feelings YOU believe in most, create the strongest energy.

Here is a Daily Prayer that with the divine guidance of God, I wrote for myself. Read it and use it as you desire.

Remember, my friend, the power lies within you...it is now time to use its fullest potential. "Physician, Heal Thyself."

—R.J.C.

*   *   *   *   *

DAILY PRAYER

This day is a day of balance. I am completely aware of my body and all its needs.
Love is my guiding light...
For love is what manifests inside me, and outside of me.
I am a ray of white light shining upon my life, and the life of others.
Make the inside like the outside, one in the same,
Union of the three, for that is peace...
For I am eternal, immortal, universal, and infinite.
I see only beauty and strength in every moment of my life.
In every breath I take, I feel the law of the universe run through my soul,
And it supports me every step of the way...
May the energy of the day strengthen and radiate the white light that I...
The "I AM" of God...surround myself with.
And may the energy of this light bring rebuilding

And peace...so be it.
I ask for the power for the union...
Of my mind, body, and spirit!

Amen.

Whoever reads these words. . .may you be at peace.

Russell John Carlton

THE UNIVERSAL LAW OR GOD FORCE WITHIN YOU

Creating energy for yourself through the Universal Law is not simply a matter of wishing for things. You must realize that YOU have the power WITHIN YOU. Once you have achieved this goal, you are that much closer to realizing your potential as a human being.
"TO MAKE THE OUTSIDE LIKE THE INSIDE... ONE AND THE SAME..."
Whatever your thoughts are manifesting, whatever you believe in, you eventually become and have.

As an individual, you must explore your thoughts and decide what you are indeed manifesting. As you are reading this, you are creating thoughts; they are powerful, and manifest themselves in the outward.

The Law of the Universe does not discriminate. The universe receives your energy and delivers diamonds or plain rocks to you, depending on what kinds of thoughts you are thinking, and how much energy you put into the manifestation.

The Universal Law, or Living Spirit, is unlimited. This

force is within you. Therefore, what you are is also unlimited.

Each person is responsible for his own evolution. Each pulls himself toward the circumstances experienced in life. Good fortune is not merely a gift from God; it is a part of WHAT YOU ARE, which is GOD.

The more you get in touch with the Universal Law within you, the more you are in touch with your reality around you. Everything and everyone becomes a symbol and strength to you.

As you watch your new awareness grow, you see that YOU ARE RESPONSIBLE for what you are. Everything around you expresses your energy.

Getting in tune with yourself and your surroundings, is the key to your Spiritual Unfoldment.

What you are has great power. Its energy oscillates and reflects the amount of Living Spirit or God Force that you express. The more YOU ACCEPT RESPONSIBILITY, the more energy you will have, and the greater your expectations and manifestations.

—R.J.C.

*   *   *   *   *

THE POWER OF HOLISTIC HEALTH

"Inside of us, there is a personal journey each takes in his own unique way." It is a reminder of the unity of all life and the essential oneness of all religions.

Each of us is on a unique and precious journey. Healing is nothing more than taking care of ourselves on this journey— a journey of cleansing the Body, Mind, and Soul.

Holistic health represents the acceptance of our entire reality—being in our bodies, owning our feelings, attitudes, and beliefs, being open to relationships and changes, and being responsible for every thought, deed, and condition we are involved in.

The way to Holistic Health is getting in touch with oneself completely. To know who you are and where you are going. To know where you came from, and to rediscover the knowledge we once all possessed and manifested.

Hear your name being called, my friend. Ascend to the unascended and there you will discover Peace in yourself and the World.

With a clear mind, we can learn to recover from excesses. We need to allow ourselves the opportunity to rest, reflect, and most important, rejuvenate—and come to terms with the behavior that was originally responsible for our disease.

If we take the time to review our lives, we will come to see the picture which we are painting. With each stroke of the brush, we slowly see before our eyes our own creation. When we come to understand our place in the cosmos, we can begin to enjoy our divine role, become creative in our performance, and at long last, become FREE OF FEAR.

The choice is yours, for we are all creators on this plane of existence. The choice that lies in front of you now is the choice of healing your Mind, Body, and Soul.

Allow yourself to feel the emotions you're going to feel, for to feel is merely to allow yourself to love yourself. Remember through allowing yourself to feel, YOU MUST also allow yourself to LET GO of these feelings of Pain, Fear, and Anger. Most of all, we need to find love and express LOVE.

Often, as we become better acquainted with who we are and where we have come from, we experience seemingly regressive needs, and release old anger and sadness. If we can let go of these, without shame or embarrassment, our grateful, joyful side will be freed as well.

An emotional clearing is like a storm, purifying the environment and nurturing the Earth. A feeling of illness is like a gathering of storm clouds, an accumulation of energy that has not yet begun to flow, and should be released.

Now is the time to see yourself strong; surround yourself with all the love and support you need. Realize that with every breath you take, the Law of the Universe is going to support you every step of the way. Believe that the energy you are investing in yourself at this time of need, will be rewarded; your body will respond to the Love you are giving it.

A powerful healing meditation is to let every thought be a prayer, asking not "Let my will be done," but "Thy will be done." This is the co-creative process made manifest.

An aimless life is a miserable life. Direct yourself on the Holistic path and reach for the stars...and be sure you believe that you will grab them!

"I ask for the power of THE UNION...of my MIND, BODY, AND SPIRIT."

Seek and you shall find, my friend. With the power of love I give thanks for all the guidance I have received.

God Bless You.

—R.J.C.

*   *   *   *   *

BLUE MOON TRILOGY

Eve of Conception—Dawning of A New Age—A Glorious
Revelation

("Blue Moon Trilogy" decorates a wall at the Odin Street underpass across from the Hollywood Bowl, and is dedicated to the AIDS crisis and opportunity, to the New Age, and the transformation in the life of the artist, Russell J. Carlton.)[1]

---

[1] "Russell Carlton: Seeing is Believing," interview by Dennis Colby, in *EDGE Magazine*, Los Angeles, California, June 10, 1987. Reprinted with permission of publisher.

QUESTION: I've read descriptions of Blue Moon Trilogy's three panels. May I have their meaning in your own words?

ANSWER: The first panel shows a comet. It's called *Eve of Conception*. This comet is coming just before something great is about to happen. I relate it to awareness. When AIDS hit us, there was much fear and hysteria. But also an awareness started to overtake us to make us realize who we are, and what we are doing. The comet is coming. Some of us realize the significance of events like the gay bashings. They show that these people would put us into concentration camps, if they could. We must realize that fear and ignorance govern these people. Their way is not going to solve anything, but only make matters worse.

The middle panel, *Dawning of a New Age*, shows the comet as landed and headed towards the moon. This portrays a new energy we are tapping. The third panel, *A Glorious Revolution*, shows the alignment of the comet and the moon, a symbol of a newly realized harmony of mind, spirit, and body.

When people go through all the discord and replace the fear with love, they enter a glorious revelation. Together they will realize they can put down their barriers and join hands and say, "We're going to wipe this out together."

If we all work to find the answers, we'll find them faster. Our sexuality is different but we're all the same, we have the same emotions, we all laugh, we can all listen to the same song and feel the same things. In time, this world will be a much better place when this is understood

The earth is so beautiful just the way it is. We get caught up in trying to change it to make our mark. If we simply let things be and realize what everything is, we will get through this crisis together. We will find the answers and find ourselves on a higher level of understanding.

SPIRITUAL REFLECTIONS OF THE ARTIST

I. EVE OF CONCEPTION
II. DAWNINGS OF A NEW AGE
III. A GLORIOUS REVELATION

In this last decade, people have in increasing numbers turned to alternatives to reduce the chance of dis-ease. People are beginning to realize that without their health they have nothing. People in general are starting to reevaluate their lifestyles and are taking more responsibility for themselves— their actions, their health.

We are becoming aware of our environment and not letting it control our destiny. A new awareness that health and happiness must start within ourselves is beginning to spread.

I refer to this new awareness as our "EVE OF CONCEP-TION." AIDS has truly given urgency to this new awareness. In reality, AIDS does not discriminate; anyone or any group of people can be stricken.

Lack of knowledge has sent many of us into a nose dive of hysteria. For many of us, the unknown instills too much fear for us to face the future. So hostility has been born from our ignorance of these new questions. We see hostility towards the victims of the dis-ease, the gay community at large, the government, the world we live in, but most of all towards ourselves. The fear is too much for many of us to consciously bear.

We have started to see a mass consciousness movement, and this is good. The ignorance is being turned around and doors to SELF-DISCOVERY, SUPPORT, and LOVE are being opened. People are starting to experience LOVE on many new levels and thereby they are turning the odds around.

Before us all is "THE DAWNING OF A NEW AGE." People are becoming aware of their bodies in a new way, their minds, and spirituality. We are experiencing the wonderful bodies we live in and understanding the tremendous healing powers we all possess. Our bodies are our temples and within these temples happiness, health, and peace can be found.

"A GLORIOUS REVELATION" is taking place right now. We are reaching out our hands for others to join us. The more we all unite, the more quickly we will find the answers we all seek to heal the dilemma we face. WE ARE ALL ONE, and by joining together in love, nothing will get in the way of this tremendous healing force.

*　　　*　　　*　　　*　　　*

AUTHORS' COMMENTS: ABOUT FASTING AND JUICES

There is an entire literature on fasting. Interested persons should read one of these books: *Fasting Can Save Your Life, Fasting for Renewal of Life,* or *The Science and Fine Art of Fasting*— all by Dr. Herbert M. Shelton, principal founder in our day of the Natural Hygiene movement.

No, "Hygiene" does not refer to cleanliness, as we know it. It comes from the Greek goddess of health, Hygeia, and the word hygiea means health or soundness of body. Even our dictionaries define "hygiene" as "the science of health and its maintenance."

Carrot juice is extremely perishable. It should be freshly squeezed in a juicer at home and used immediately, for best results.

Beta-Carotene, the substance which makes carrots orange, is found to lower the risk of cancer. Beta-Carotene is also found to a lesser degree in sweet potatoes, yams, and green vegetables.

No harm and only good can come to a person on the fast (actually, a diet of carrot juice and herbs) Russell John Carlton was on.

There is a case, famous in the natural health movement, of Mrs. Ferraro of Monrovia, California. Some years ago, she was near death of leukemia. A friend, who knew the value of carrot juice, urged her to consume one gallon of fresh carrot juice per day, and consume no other food. She agreed to try it, and was totally healed. In gratitude, she and her family started a company processing and selling carrot juice, calling it, "Liquid Gold". Ferraro's Juices in Monrovia continues to thrive.

Dr. Norman Walker, who lived to 109, was a pioneer in "juice therapy." He wrote books on the subject, and invented the "Norwalk Juicer."

The literature on fasting states that a fatality might occur if a person goes on a total fast (no food at all), for a long period of time, and unsupervised. He is then not fasting, but starving himself. It is not generally known that a person on a total fast does not feel the hunger that a person feels when on a juice diet. Also, rest is essential when one is abstaining entirely from food. A knowledgeable professional who is accustomed to supervising fasts, should oversee a total fast.

Dr. Paavo Airola, nutritionist and author, recommended juice fasts (really juice diets), rather than total fasts. The Natural Hygiene movement can tell many true stories of various acute and chronic diseases being healed with total fasts (abstinence from food), but strongly urges that these be supervised. The body must be monitored daily for changes.

The motto of Natural Hygiene is "Health care is self care."

THE TRUTH ABOUT SUGAR

The valuable mineral calcium is lost in refining sugar cane. When refined sugar, or sucrose, enters the digestive tract, it combines with the calcium there, forming calcium saccharate. This new product is thrown off by the body, thus robbing it of calcium, an indispensable mineral in maintaining strong, healthy teeth.

It is better to eat natural sweets: fruits, dates, and honey, the latter two in moderation.

A large number of researchers have studied the effects of sugar on the human body and have definitely proven that it is a dangerous killer! Dr. John Yudkin, M.D., calls it "The Quiet Killer" that can cause heart disease, diabetes, ulcers, and other often-fatal diseases.

Dr. Yudkin writes.... "My research on coronary disease has convinced me beyond doubt that sugar plays a considerable part in this terrifying modern epidemic.... If only a fraction of what is already known about the effects of sugar were to be revealed, the use of that substance would promptly be banned."

According to J. I. Rodale, sugar robs the body of vitamin B (thiamine), and also is detrimental to the mind, adversely affecting the bloodstream and then the brain.

When hyperactive children have sugar excluded from their diets, they become "angels." Their problems lessen greatly, and their learning ability is greatly enhanced.

RECOMMENDED READING

(1)   *Natural Health, Sugar and the Criminal Mind* by J. I. Rodale, a Pyramid Book, 1968. This book is a startling, thought-provoking study of the life-and-death role of nutrition and how it affects social problems.

(2)   *Crime & Diet: The Macrobiotic Approach* by Michio Kushi, Japan Publications, USA, 1987. As incidence of crime and delinquency rises, more and more clinical and statistical evidence points to diet as cause and solution. In this break-through book Kushi explains how many physical conditions are linked to behavioral problems. He tells why those physical conditions are diet induced, and how they can be cured nutritionally. Case histories of dietary solutions to mental conditions are presented.

(3)   *Sugar Blues* by William Dufty, Warner Books, 1975. It tells about the hidden dangers of eating sugar—and also of its relationship to obesity.

(4)   *Lick the Sugar Habit* by Nancy Appleton, Ph. D., Warner Books, 1985. Explains how sugar addiction upsets the entire chemistry of the body and devastates the immune system. The book is a forceful attack on a lifestyle and eating habits that can lead to degenerative diseases. The author tells how an excess of refined sugar is linked to heart disease, diabetes, food allergies, calcium loss, tooth decay, periodontal diseases, osteoporosis, hypoglycemia, arthritis, cancer, headaches, asthma, etc. She shows that the U. S. is a nation of sugarholics, slaves and victims of sugar. We consume on the average more than 130 pounds of sugar and sweeteners a year, per person.

(5)   *Why Your Child is Hyperactive* by Ben Feingold, M.D., Random House, N.Y., N.Y., 1975.

(6)   *Sweet and Dangerous* by John Yudkin, M.D., Bantam Books, 1972.

Niro Asistent

To look at Niro Asistent, you would believe her to be a totally feminine woman. Her short blond hair falls softly about her face and her eyes have a gentle expression. She seems the embodiment of femininity. Yet beneath this soft exterior, she is firm with the unswerving firmness of knowing herself, what she is about, and what she wishes to accomplish in this world. She is a very compassionate woman, a gentle and lovely woman, but a determined one. She is working for goals which she feels are worthwhile, and nothing is going to shake her or turn her from her path. Her hardness is determination and strength to move along the path of spiritual enlightenment— and to help others with every facet of her many capabilities.

She understands loneliness, beauty, and that quality of the human spirit that makes all mankind worthy of respect and love. She is very human, for she has felt panic, rejection, and periodic love, and transcended them. She has learned all the lessons contained in her own encounters, reaping an awareness of life and her relation to it—and of the needs of man and her rapport with those needs. Such is Niro, resident of New York state—a loving, responsive, gentle, and dedicated woman.

In the Rajneesh Ashram in Oregon, Niro and Nado met. Here they became lovers. Here, they studied, learned, and translated their knowledge into their way of life. Rajneesh was constantly advocating "safe sex," so at one point in their relationship, Niro and Nado started practicing "safe sex." Unknown to them at the time, it was too late.

Niro Asistent's Adventure

In early September of 1985 in the Ashram, Nado and I went to a medical doctor, whom we knew by the religious name of Swami Pragyan. He tested us both for AIDS. We both tested positive; Nado was highly positive. The test used was the ELISA. Nado had tested so highly, it was not deemed necessary to give him the Western Blot.

Nado was bisexual; he did not discuss it, but I knew. Even though in the Ashram we were very informed about AIDS, somehow it was not my reality. It was a fiction. It was something that was "out there." Something we were concerned about in an uninvolved way. I never even considered it as something that would enter my life.

Our first reaction was denial, then panic. We went immediately to our own doctor, Dr. Cairns, in New York. He was wonderful. He said he would not even put it on our record. This was in 1985, which was the year of the beginning wave of panic about AIDS. There was worry about losing employment or insurance, since insurance companies were refusing to pay for the high costs of treating AIDS. Our doctor advised us at this time to go to the Suffolk Health Department, and assured us that our anonymity would be preserved, as they dealt with numbers in identifying recipients of the test.

We were still panicking and wanted a verification of the illness as soon as possible, so we went instead to the Red Cross. We gave blood and filled out the questionnaire. At this point, one of the Red Cross workers said, "If something is in your blood, it will take six months for the information to reach you."

Our odyssey then took us to the Suffolk Health Department. It was then the beginning of October. We got the results in mid-November, 1985. We were given both tests at this time, the ELISA and the Western Blot. My lover's results were very high; mine were not so high, but the symptoms were catching up with me. I was very tired with fever most of the time, and my body was starting to deteriorate. I was losing much weight, but I was happy about that. Most of my life I have been overweight. I also had diarrhea, candidiasis, and thrush.

Nado tested positive in September, and I tested positive in November of 1985. For that entire time, from the period of his positive results and the results of my test, I was in total denial and anger. It was not even a question. I just said, "I will not have that." Even though I had certain symptoms that indicated AIDS, I would not put them together to draw that terrible conclusion. I was just exhausted, I told myself, because I had worked too much. I was not eating right. My body is reacting to being ignored and mistreated. I am merely physically rundown and weak.

It was strange, while I was waiting in the car for my appointment to get the results of the testing, I kept looking at nature around me. Nado and I had driven to the Center together, arriving early. It was a beautiful day, and I was enjoying the serenity. Then, about twenty minutes before I was to go into the building the thought reached me, "Stop fooling yourself; you know you will test positive. When you come out of that building with the results, you will be a different person." So I was prepared for the diagnosis, as prepared as one could ever be. It was a sort of clicking inside me, and I knew; it was a desperate knowing.

My first reaction was one of sadness, then anger. All aspects of the media—newspapers, magazines, radio, and television—were completely negative and destructive, denying the right to hope in their unequivocal statements that the disease was fatal, that there was no cure. I was filled with anger by this, but I accepted it.

At the time of the testing we were given a booklet containing instructions as to what steps we should take to postpone our date with death, but I didn't even read them. I accepted death as the ultimate destination, and just lived day by day. I set up my own rules for living and followed them without deviation. They were simple.

Throughout my life, I have been a seeker, searching for the meaning of life and for spiritual fulfillment. Under Rajneesh, I had learned a meditation which I now brought into my life and did every single day. The meditation lasts an hour. The first thirty minutes, you hum—not only with your voice, but with a vibration. You realign your breath all the way from the third chakra up, so that the vibration takes place at the base of the nose. You breathe very deeply, but in a relaxed way. You are sitting in the lotus position with your spine very stretched, and you are very centered. In the second stage, the music changes—you have a tape. The music for the first thirty minutes is Tibetan bells; this supports the opening of the chakra. When the music changes, you allow your hands to move in a circle with your palms upright. You don't hum anymore, and you keep your eyes closed. You focus on giving your energy to the universe. Then, after seven and a half minutes of that, the music changes and you do a circle going inward with the palm down, and you focus on receiving from the universe. For the last part of the meditation, you lie down. This is a wonderful meditation. I give it out now to help people. I feel it helped me so much. Now, I wouldn't be without it.

The other thing I did was take long walks on the beach. This was very helpful. It was as if I wanted to—had a need to—get back to nature. I have always been a doer. I was never really one to enjoy quiet walks along the beach or in the park. Now they are a part of my life that I love.

But these two activities that I brought into my life on a regular basis after I learned of the positive diagnosis were not considered cures. I did not even think of a cure. The cure—or what the medical profession knew about AIDS and its cure—was contained in a booklet given us after the diagnosis. It had the telephone number of Sunny Brook Research University and many pages about this illness.

But to tell you the truth, I didn't want to hear about it. I just wanted to run out of the health department building. I didn't have any questions; I just wanted to be by myself. My conviction at that time was, "Oh, I have only two years to live." I have never used drugs—but it was as if I was "stoned." I was totally frozen. I kept saying to myself, "I will not have any emotion. I will not cry. I will not talk." I felt like a robot.

I did not know how to behave upon being given that kind of news. I didn't know what to do, so I started straightening my affairs in a legal way, for my two children. I started to complete many things that were unfinished. I threw away many papers, and those I kept I went over carefully to be sure everything was there, and that my children would understand them. I got the best life insurance I could get. All those details were really my major concern for three weeks. That's all I did. I didn't even open the booklet I had received from the Suffolk County Health Department.

I didn't ever really think about healing. Dr. Cairns gave me the name of a famous doctor at Sunny Brook University, and I called his office one day. The lady who answered asked what my symptoms were. When I told her, she said, "You are not sick enough. You will have to wait two months for an appointment."

"To hell with that," I said. "I won't sit here waiting for two months."

I had heard of people running to Mexico to do various things to find a cure, but I absolutely wouldn't do that. I didn't want to read one thing about AIDS. I didn't look at the news on TV; I didn't read the newspaper. I tried to isolate myself from the media and its negative publicity.

What I had heard and read on AIDS, I did not believe, and it was creating a great deal of anger in me. So I decided to isolate myself from the media.

When I was a child, I was subject to much illness. I learned at that time how to manipulate illness. I also developed an instinctive distrust of doctors. As a child, when I was sick, the only thing I wanted was just to be taken care of; doctors never do that. I wanted loving care at home. Because of my childhood experiences, I learned to trust my own intuition, and I always tried to heal myself first. I don't go to a doctor right away unless it's for some specific need for the children. With this illness, when my fever went up, I took Excedrin or Tylenol. In my approach to medication, I tend to the holistic approach, but I'm also very practical. I will never deny using it when a specific medication seems to be the answer.

Prior to my illness, my lifestyle was regular, because of my religious leanings. I was center coordinator in one of the larger Rajneesh meditation centers on the East coast. I was practicing spiritual therapy, leading meditation, and I had had training in breath therapy and balancing. In addition, I was fortunate enough to have a job on a beautiful estate. This also contributed to the regularity of my lifestyle.

At the time of my diagnosis, I would not say that I was promiscuous. I was very faithful to my lover, although there were periods when I felt rejected by him as a woman. Once, during a period like this, it was so painful that I met with one of my friends. He was also a disciple of Bhagwan Rajneesh, and he was also practicing "safe sex." While Nado was my lover, this man was the only other partner I had. In the middle of intercourse, we really wanted to kiss each other. Then we said, "No, we will follow the rules." Thank God we did, because after that I found that I was HIV positive. Six months later we spoke by telephone and said, "Thank God, we followed the rules." He was concerned and wanted to be tested right away; he tested negative.

Because of this experience, I feel that "safe sex" is safe. Maybe it's not foolproof, but it is a protection. "Safe sex" isn't easy. My lover and I were practicing it because Rajneesh had emphasized the need to do this. We made fun about it, asking each other all the time, "How's your love life?" We were using condoms, and we were not French kissing. When you have had a normal relationship and suddenly you cannot French kiss, it is very difficult and frustrating. French kissing was one part of our sexual behavior. Following the rules of "safe sex" for us meant a lot of willingness, a lot of love, and a lot of will power.

There are a few things a person can do to protect himself or herself from the AIDS virus. Of course, one must practice "safe sex." Another, be sure where the needle is coming from in a blood transfusion, and if possible, where the blood is coming from. The world of drugs is a risky one, and filled with Persons With AIDS. One must be careful with sex, and also with the interchange of bodily fluids and blood.

In addition, I feel that this virus could have been spread by the research laboratories. It could have been a by-product of something that got away. This thought has been in my mind lately.

On February 4, 1986, Nado died. I am not really familiar with Nado's disease record. I know that he was reared in the Far East, and that he had many endemic illnesses as a child. He didn't ever have malaria. During his adult life, he was strong and very, very healthy. I know he was in the hospital once before our relationship, but I do not know what medications or drugs, if any, he received. Nado was a dancer. He had spent his life caring for his body, its health and beauty of perform-ance. He was very healthy, and now he is dead.

When I was fighting to turn the disease around, I said, "Nado, let's do it together." His answer was, "You know I'm doing just exactly what I choose to do." He was very clear. He died very complete. He was also a poet and the last six months of his life, he wrote more than during all his previous life. He seemed to be exploding with creativity, and he was totally happy just being creative in his writing. He had no interest in my forms of healing. His healing was happening on another plane. Death was his choice, but I chose to live.

I feel that Nado's death was avoidable. The last two days before his death, we were very close to each other, because we were both HIV positive Then, for me, tremendous anger started to come. He didn't want to talk about it, and I wanted to talk about it. He gently withdrew. Nado always said he would die at forty-two. His former wife told me that she remembered his saying that. He died because he felt it was the time for him to die. I really had a hard time with his answer—and his death—but it helps me often today in my work.

Now, when I meet people who really feel they want to leave this life, I give them some space. I have attachments to them and desire that they get well, but I must give them the right of choice to be where they are, to make their decisions. I must support them, and if necessary, I must let them go without anger. I learned that from Nado.

The gay community was heavily stricken by the AIDS virus. When Nado was alive, I was fearful of the gay commu-nity, fearful of rejection, but after his death I found them very loving and accepting. I had much compassion for them, because they come from a place of anger. Anger itself can create disease. They need to be educated and helped. This situation is leading me into a new life. Now, I go and speak and inform.

I have dedicated my life to the SHARE Foundation and other organizations involved with and supporting PWA's. I created the SHARE Foundation with two gay friends. It means Self-healing, AIDS-Related Experiment. It is a non-profit organization under the umbrella of the Northern Lights with Charles Baier, Victor Phillips from Northern Lights and Sally Fisher. At present, I am doing a lot of fund-raising for People With AIDS. The project for SHARE is to create a residential center. We have people who are stuck in the hospital. Some are penniless, homeless, workless. They have nothing, and they have no place to go. So we are focusing on supporting them.

Another part of my life is dealing with PWA's, so they can live with the issue. Because I have the training and the personal experience, I can relate to them. Unfortunately, what I observe is many people with good intentions hammering at PWA's with only prophecies and good advice.

AIDS is considered to be a venereal disease. I realize that it is also transmitted by the blood and other bodily fluids. It is believed to infect those who have a health record of previous venereal diseases. I have not had any venereal diseases.

Before my life with Nado, I was promiscuous. I was also bisexual. However, I do not feel that my lifestyle was in any way involved in my getting this illness. Through the influence of the Ashram, Nado and I were at the time of diagnosis practicing "safe sex" as mentioned, but I feel I was infected by him during our relationship prior to this practice. I have never smoked cigarettes or marijuana. I do not take drugs; I have not had any transfusions or antibiotics. After accepting Nado as my lover, I was faithful. He was bisexual, and must have become infected with the virus during one of those periods when he was rejecting me and having sex with a male lover. There is no question in my mind as to how I got the disease. I received it from my bisexual lover.

After those first three weeks, which were disastrous, I began to live a normal life again. My friends and family were very supportive of me. My children were wonderful to me. Puja, one of my friends, came and lived with me. She didn't really help me in any physical sense. She was just there for me. It was comforting, and important for me. I did not tell my family, who are still in Europe, about my illness until much later.

There is a psychological aspect of AIDS. I felt it. It seemed as if I were a total outcast. It was the feeling that I was different, the feeling that I had a burden on me, that AIDS was something to be ashamed of. I was not ashamed of myself, but I assumed people would reject me because I had AIDS, would avoid me, or look down on me.

There was also the psychological effect of the media. They had stamped their belief on the public via every public method of communication saying "all PWA's will die." I totally embodied that belief. That was my reality. I was not even questioning it. I mention this again, because it had so much influence on the way I responded to the disease when I began to live a normal life. I made my decision consciously. I would not go to a doctor for treatment or to a hospital. My plan was this: when my body would begin to fall apart totally, then I would shorten the process. I consider this different from suicide. While there was life, I would continue to live it as I always had—in a spiritual way, seeking answers.

One of the answers to my way of life was a new diet. I had begun to realize that my diet was not good. Although I was a vegetarian, I was not eating properly. I was living on cookies, chocolates, and ice cream. I consumed no meat, no fish, no chicken, but that didn't mean my diet was a good one. I came to realize this and changed my food habits completely.

I went on a drastic diet. I have been overweight most of my life, and I went to a clinic for losing weight called "Health Management." The diet consisted of a protein powder with an egg white base. I did not associate this with a step in healing, but I followed the diet extremely seriously. The only food I took was the protein powder and the accompanying vitamins. I had all the necessary vitamins, minerals, and protein required on a daily basis. I suppose you could say that I detoxified my body in a way similar to the effect of a fast, because I followed this regime for three and a half months, and I excreted many bodily toxins.

But I can honestly say that I did not think of healing. I did not think of getting well, only of living my life to the fullest—whatever was left of it.

My lifestyle changed as a result of the illness, because my requirements seemed to change. There was an urge to get back to nature. My meditation became very important. I would not let the day go by without it, and also walks on the beach and in the park. These were healing therapies which I failed to recognize as such at first. After one month of meditation, about two months after hearing the diagnosis, I started to feel really strong. The diarrhea stopped. I thought it was because of my diet. I wasn't feeling so tired. My energy level went up. I felt healthy. I was living with the seasons. It was winter, so I was resting a great deal. I was eating well, and I was seeing only friends who were really still loving. I was not seeking health, or a cure. I was reading a great deal, but not books on health and related subjects. I read a book on Zen and meditation. All the books I read were spiritual in nature.

Without realizing it, my character was changing. I was much more at peace. I didn't feel pushed any more. I didn't have to accomplish anything. From always being a doer, I suddenly became somebody who could go with the flow. With the walks, and listening to beautiful music, my life became very simple. I wasn't focusing on getting well, just on totally doing what I was doing. It had to be total. I was very happy when I was walking on the beach. I was looking at the ocean, thinking of the ocean, responding to the ocean totally in my way. I was much happier than I had ever been before. I had a craving to be in contact with nature completely. So while my life was simple, it was very fulfilling.

In February, I was walking on the beach when I received

a flash, an insight that told me, "You're healed. You're fine. You're healed!"

It was like a voice inside me. I remember that moment very, very clearly.

Right away, after that, I called the Suffolk County Medical Department for a retesting. I couldn't get an appointment until the end of March, but I went then, and they did three tests. I got the answer the beginning of May. Test results: totally negative. Everybody was amazed. I showed no sign of the virus.

The same tests were taken that had been taken before. Only now, the results were negative. The lady who was there at the time I tested positive started to treat me as if I were suddenly very fragile and going to die in two hours. The lady who was there when I tested negative was completely amazed. They took a lot of blood, and then they took some more tests.

Finally, I said, "You know I'm here now. I don't want to be anonymous anymore. We really have a relationship. Give my full name to Albany because the Center where everything is happening is Albany." The Suffolk County Health Department was asking for more and more blood. I really wanted to know what they were doing with it, and what they had to say, but I have never been told. I probably have phoned over thirty times, and still I have no report of what they have done or are doing with my blood. I said to the lady, "Put me in touch, because people need to know about my recovery." I was so excited that I told her I was alone. It's only lately when I'm with Anita, Bill, and George—and plenty of other people who are in remission—that I realize that I am no longer alone.

In New York, the gay community opened to me with no reservations. I feel totally loved and accepted there. I feel the difference, and I just love them. I love the way we work together, and I'm very grateful. I still have my old friends, but I don't see them so often, because I work so much. Now I have all those new friends. I'm very close with Anita, and I've known her only three months. I love her. We're like sisters. And Will and George are key people in my life, and I didn't know them six months ago.

I realize that I am not the only one to survive AIDS. The statement of the media is not true—AIDS is not 100% fatal. I say this although I know that many Persons With AIDS do die as a result of their infection.

Through my work with SHARE (Self-Healing, AIDS Related Experiment), I have come in contact with many people. Some don't want to live, and they die. Some want to live, and they die. Some want to live, and they do live. I feel that some of the deaths are the result of the body's being too far gone, whether from the infection, or from the body's condition when the infection was contracted. I really believe that some of the Persons With AIDS die because in the process of doing everything required to achieve a cure, they really find what they have to learn in this lifetime. It's through that incredible seeking process, that they really get what they need to get, and they are ready to die.

I don't believe these people do anything wrong that causes them to die. I think if we would work with those people we would find that at a deep level somewhere, they choose to leave the body at that time. People respond with anger when I say that, but I know in my guts that's the truth. You know I've been doing metaphysical work and spiritual work for AIDS, so for me this is my life. Of course, if you would take somebody from the street who has never approached that concept, you would create a lot of anger. I have much compassion for that, and try to give them space to know what is their choice. But I know they don't do anything wrong, absolutely not. They forget to love and accept themselves unconditionally.

It sounds horrible, but the ones who don't make it, yet have expressed a wish to live, do not really have a total desire to do so. Somewhere, on some level, they want to die, even though they do all the things that they can to create a cure. They are not really committed to live. You know it's one thing to live, but it's the total "yes!" to living that counts. I am expressing only my feeling.

When I give lectures, I always tell people, "Getting sick was hard for me; getting to the point where I got sick was very tough. Healing myself hasn't been easy, but it's been natural." You know sometimes people do everything, but they are doing and not allowing or "letting." Yet, one can't make a general statement. It's different in every case, and I know that. I'm working with one person now whose commitment to live is extremely fragile. The person goes back and forth all the time. The final decision will be his.

What these people do who die is not wrong. It is just their choice. No one can say why one person will die and another will not. It is only the person who is going through the process of living or dying who can answer the question of "why."

My choice was to live. I was talking to one of my friends, just after Nado died. I said, "It's amazing. I feel I have much guilt and much pain, and much love." What came up in the discussion was my knowing that I can create the disease in me again very easily.

Last week, I was working with a group and I realized for the first time that lately I don't have a great desire to be in my body. My lover's on the other side; he is not here anymore. Oddly enough, I'm having new tests. I'm having tests all the time, because last week the night sweats and sore throat returned. I ran to my doctor, Dr. Cairns, and he said, "You know you don't have any swollen glands or anything like that." Then he added, "You have too much to do. You can't get sick again, Niro."

Dr. Cairns is a wonderful man. He's a seeker himself, looking for the spiritual. I told him, "I will not seek for any cure. I'm going to meditate."

He simply said, "Keep on doing the good work." He

was wonderful. He didn't try to force any of his opinions on me.

My lifestyle changed, too, with Nado's death. I am no longer sexually active at all. It's not that the desire is no longer there. I loved Nado, and my pain needs to heal. I have not yet been able to find a partner to whom I can feel close enough— someone with whom I can feel open enough to accept him as a new partner.

There are so many ways in which my lifestyle has changed. I am no longer involved with Rajneesh. He was my master, and it was wonderful being a disciple, but now that is complete. It is the past. I am no longer involved with the organization as a coordinator; I am devoting my time totally to PWA's. I do not do any writing, because English is not my native language, but I lecture and speak on AIDS in New York. I am devoted to this cause and am very busy.

My income is another thing. I no longer have the job I had when I was tested positive, so I need some kind of income. The work I'm doing does not as yet provide that, but it's going to have to provide my income. I may have to ask for support. I do not doubt that I will get help. I'm into the project, and I'm willing to move mountains. The AIDS programs are my life.

You know, we all have AIDS. One has it in his body, and one has it in his mind. We all suffer from the illness. Just look at the media. There is not one newspaper or magazine that doesn't have an article on AIDS weekly or daily. We are all suffering because of the media. People are fearful of even mentioning AIDS. It's an issue that they don't bring up. It's in everything—politics, economics. And the fear, it's in everyone! There is an epidemic of fear. So when I fund-raise, I create the opportunity for people to give money—so they can object to that doom, so they can feel responsible, so they can heal themselves. Naturally, they're concerned, and giving that energy we call money is a very good outlet. I approach everybody with the issue. People can give me three dollars or three thousand—I don't care. The circle enlarges. We are on the move. The moment people are willing to give, something happens. There is a flow.

Diet is very important, but what works for me might not work for someone else. Listen to that inner voice, trust it and follow it. I love miso soup and broccoli, but I will not go to other people and tell them to eat miso soup and broccoli. For another person, it could be sunflower seeds and for someone else, it could be strawberries. Diet is important, but there is no one perfect diet for everyone. Each person is unique and needs his own special diet.

My diet has changed because my thinking has changed, because my way of looking at life is different. Life is the greatest gift. Before, I took life for granted.

I eat very little junk food now. I'm still a vegetarian, but now I eat more high quality vegetables.

I would like to have a residence system set up quickly, and become 100% busy with that. Right now, I am not thinking of a community. We have the need to create a place for people to be, to have space, to make their choice. We also have emergency situations to take care of. These are my future plans: to aid the people and to influence the media so they see the positive aspects of AIDS.

Since I was tested positive, I have not yet read a book on AIDS. I was helped by books I read, but they were not specifically on AIDS. I read and utilized a great book called *Creative Visualization* by Shakti Gawain. Another book that helped me was *The Book of Wisdom* by Rajneesh.

I consider this disease the greatest blessing of my life. In photography, there is a liquid where you put in the picture that is to be revealed. This disease has revealed what was inside me. It has always been inside me, but now it is revealed to me. I have discovered the person that I am. This knowledge has helped me be more capable of helping others. It has helped me in the work I have chosen to do. Among other things, it taught me the value of my inner strength, my inner voice. It gave me the strength to trust my intuition, to listen to what was happening inside me, and to say "no" to the rest of the planet.

I have learned the importance of turning the other cheek with AIDS. The goal of my life is to change the doom energy. I want to keep spreading the love and receiving the love, and spreading the love and receiving the love....

Everyone is different. Everyone has his own way of life and path, and must seek his own cure. I want to be supportive, but there is one bit of advice which I feel everyone can benefit from. It is simply "Love yourself unconditionally."

I am so busy now, working with SHARE, Northern Lights, the Healing Circle, and Samuel Kirshner. He is wonderful. What he is doing is incredible! I keep in touch now with the Gay Men's Health Crisis. I go to the Bailey House, which is a hospice. Anywhere I feel that it's needed for me to go, I go. This is my life; this is my choice.

WHAT NIRO ASISTENT DID

• She lived one day at a time.

• She was willing to accept death, but did everything she could to live.

• She believed that meditation would help her, and she used it for her healing.

• She learned to live with the seasons. In winter, she would rest more. In the summer, she devoted long hours to walking on the beach and otherwise getting back to Nature.

• She listened to the rhythm of the environment around her.

• She did not run away from her problem, but decided to confront it, head on.

• She did not read newspapers; she did not watch television. She stayed away from all negative influences.

• She knew that the media are being manipulated by the establishment, and that there are dangerous untruths being broadcast on AIDS, causing an epidemic of fear.

• She trusted her own intuition. She learned to listen to the "still, small voice" within her.

• She made healing herself the first priority in her life.

• She early decided that she would not run around frantically to doctors, seeking a cure. She was slapped with AIDS, but did not react violently.

• She changed her junk food vegetarian diet to a wholesome one. (A person can live on "Twinkies" and Cokes, and still call himself a vegetarian!)

• Since she was overweight, she went on a special weight-loss diet.

• She started using supplements.

• She kept only friends who were loving and supportive.

• She felt that she did not have to accomplish anything.

• She believed that health is the normal state of mankind, that natural healing is easy, and that the body will cooperate with your desire to be well, if you do not interfere with it.

• She knew that AIDS IS NOT 100% FATAL, and she proved it by the reversal of her HIV-positive diagnosis.

• After her recovery, she shared her experience—how to live without fear, and how to cope with and overcome AIDS.

• She became involved with organizations. She started "S.H.A.R.E." She talked before many groups as a volunteer.

• She developed an inner strength.

• She was and is an independent spirit.

• She realized that everyone has his/her own way of life and will seek the necessary healing in a unique way. There are many paths, all of them good for someone.

• She learned to love herself unconditionally.

- Today, she experiences life as a daily, divine, precious gift.

- This was Niro's choice.

- This is Niro Asistent's life.

Postscript

Just before this book went to press Niro said to Bianca Leonardo: "**I get tested every three months, and I still test negative.** I feel fantastic! I have never felt better in my life."

(COPY OF LETTER)

September 9, 1987

To Whom It May Concern:

Niro Asistent is a warm, dedicated person who has a great commitment to help lessen the pain of those afflicted by the AIDS crisis.

Niro Asistent herself has lost a lover to AIDS and is knowledgeable about HIV infection.

Ms. Asistent has training in Gestalt therapy and maintains a private practice. She desires to work as a volunteer in the fight against AIDS. I recommend her with no hesitation to you.

Sincerely,

Philip M. Ramu, A.C.S.W.
HIV Program Coordinator
AIDS Institute
New York State Department of Health

THE FOUNDATION FOR
"THE SELF-HEALING AIDS RELATED EXPERIMENT"

S.H.A.R.E.
A Non-Profit Organization

The purpose of the Foundation is to create a center where AIDS education will be available in an environment of love and acceptance. We explore and provide alternative healing methods and encourage spiritual growth to supplement state of the art medical care.

*   *   *   *   *

NIRO ASISTENT, Director, is a woman who shares the complex experience of having been diagnosed as having ARC in November, 1985. By using methods learned through her varied training as a therapist, she has been in full remission since May, 1986. She utilizes these healing methods for S.H.A.R.E.'s course, giving to those who have AIDS or ARC, as well as those in high risk categories, the opportunity to live life fully with the disease.

S.H.A.R.E. will enable participants with AIDS or ARC, or those in high risk categories, to move beyond their limits and transform their attitudes toward the disease from victim to master. We bring forth our inner force so that it will always be accessible at any moment. Our life then becomes a challenge instead of a series of circumstances coming at us.

S.H.A.R.E. will awaken the doctor within each of us, creating a clear dialogue between the self and the body.

magnifies the warmth generated by a small group.

> Location: S.H.A.R.E.
> TRS Inc., Professional Suite
> 7 East 30th Street
> New York, NY 10016
>
> Telephone: (212) 685-2848
> Hours: 10:00 a.m.—5:00 p.m.

*   *   *   *   *

NIRO STRESSES:

The purpose for S.H.A.R.E. is taking a larger dimension. The need for a residential center in New York is crucial, so we are now focusing on that issue as a priority.

Also, those persons who are in remission are all striving to help persons who now have AIDS, especially those in hospitals who are penniless and homeless.

*   *   *   *   *

NIRO ASISTENT studied at the Institut des Sciences Sociales de Bruxelles, served in the International Red Cross from 1958 to 1961, and was an active member of the Service Civil International in Europe. She founded and directed the B.R.M.C. Meditation Center in New York from 1983 to 1985. Her training includes Gestalt therapy, transformational therapy, breath therapy, energy balancing, and Eastern meditative practices.

Daniel Turner

The San Francisco General Hospital has a varied profile with many-storied sections and sprawling one-story additions, as its growth has kept pace with the growth of a large city, one of the oldest and most beautiful cities in the West.

Daniel Turner had the unusual experience of selecting various alternative, natural therapies in a wing of this traditional medical hospital in the Mission section of San Francisco.

Not long ago, all that personified the original spirit of freedom of choice in the United States dwelt in this wing. Two types of healing experimentally co-existed side by side. The message of the staff to Daniel Turner and others in this special program was:

"This we offer you, the quintessence of our learning— our total support in whatever way we can serve you in your search for health. We give you the right to choose, as we know that each individual requires a different stimulus to initiate his own healing."

During this period, many patients who entered the hospital with fear and despair left with renewed strength, health, and new life. Unfortunately, this special program ended, and is no longer available at San Francisco General, or any other hospital, to our knowledge. But Daniel Turner was fortunate to be in this special program.

He appreciates San Francisco General, the hospital that served him when he first got AIDS and needed help. The entire staff was fine, but he remembers in particular Dr. Paul Volberding, of whom he says: "I have never had a better doctor. We didn't always agree, but he didn't put obstacles in my path. He was always there when I needed him, but he didn't censure me or criticize when I wanted to add or experiment with alternative therapies. He was a very learned doctor, but he was more than this; he was an involved, caring human being. He wanted me well and he respected my wishes."

Daniel Turner's Adventure

When I first got AIDS, I didn't know what I had. The term AIDS was not yet in use.

In December of 1981, my first two lesions appeared. By February of 1982, I had three more and was diagnosed as having Kaposi's sarcoma, a form of cancer. This was fortunately several years after my bout with hepatitis in 1975, an illness that was very traumatic for me.

Being a patient and susceptible to paranoic fears, I felt that because they didn't give me any treatment to speak of, there was none. I thought I was on my own. Psychologically, this dependence upon myself was very good for me later on.

I realized that K.S. is a form of cancer; I also knew of

people who had survived. So this was not as traumatic as my bout with hepatitis, because I was receiving treatment—not only for the K.S., but for a parasitical infection which I had at the time.

Prior to the outbreak of AIDS, there was a lot of parasitical infection in the gay community. With my amoebic infiltration, I didn't have any symptoms. It wasn't until February of 1982, when I was going through extensive testing because of other symptoms, that they discovered I had the parasites and started treatement for them.

By the end of April of 1982, my parasitical infection was gone and my K.S. had stopped proliferating. So my K. S. stabilized essentially the same time I got rid of the parasites. I thought this was significant. However, not knowing if I would remain stable, I continued chemotherapy for two more months and then went off the treatment in July of 1982. But I remained in the hospital.

In August, I started treatment with Alpha-Interferon. There were ten patients on it for eight weeks, one week on and one week off. They allowed us to sustain continual maintenance after the study. I stayed on Alpha-Interferon for five years. When I began Interferon, my K.S. became inactive and in a few months some of the lesions faded away.

For a year and a half, I took twelve grams of vitamin C a day. I also exercised; I ran and I went to the gym. Basically, I slowed down in my lifestyle, and I took care of myself!

All my life, I had considered my lifestyle a good one. When I was diagnosed with K.S., the only prior contributing factors I had were the parasitical infection and my sexual habits. So, I feel that AIDS is definitely sex-related.

I was in New York in May and June of 1981, combining business with my vacation. I assume that I was exposed at this time through sexual encounters and permissiveness.

My basic health was good. I was eating well and was on natural foods. I didn't do drugs. Aside from my sexual activity, my lifestyle was a healthy one. If I were rundown at all, it was because I was overworking, which involved late hours and a certain amount of stress.

We know that AIDS is also acquired by contact with contaminated blood, but I feel it is most commonly transmitted sexually, although even this method of infection has conditional factors. So much depends on the state of the individual's health. The way his or her body reacts to exposure results in the specifics they get. Whether they are able to fight the effect of the virus—whether the body recognizes the virus as an enemy and martials its defenses—these are all important factors. Presumably, people who are rundown and contending with other viruses or infections or the drug habit, have a difficult time contending with the virus and are more apt to succumb.

My reaction was not traumatic when I was diagnosed as having K.S. At that time, the medical profession was not using the term AIDS. It had not yet come into existence. I was fortunate in not having to deal with a disease that was "fatal." I was receiving treatment and had every hope of regaining my health.

Six months later they began to call the illness AIDS; it was as if I were being diagnosed all over again. Initially, I was reacting to a rare cancer. Now it was another story. I realized the sickness left me open to other infections.

My diagnosis was not changed, but at the same time the two symptoms being manifested were recognized by the Centers for Disease Control as AIDS. What I want to point out is that at the time I actually had AIDS, I did not have the trauma of a "fatal" illness. I did not have to contend with the media and its sensationalism. I thought I had cancer, and I thought I had a chance. I had this chance because of my earlier bout with hepatitis.

Through my experience with hepatitis, I learned to become more self-reliant. I wasn't supplanting the medical profession in my treatment, but I did realize that my healing was in part up to me. I couldn't just sit back and ask someone else to cure me. I had to become involved, too. In a sense, I had to heal myself.

The doctors declared that my liver function had returned to normal in three months, but I perpetuated the illness psychologically, holding on to it for a year. Not realizing the importance of the mind of the patient to his healing, I remained "ill." I had not been given any treatment; only rest was recommended, so I didn't understand how I could be cured. In a way I'm grateful for my hepatitis session, because I learned so much about me—not only my body but my mind and its relationship to health. Once I realized I had "nourished" my illness mentally for a year, I vowed I would never do it again.

This resolution strengthened my determination to win my battle with AIDS. I had already survived for six months, and I refused to think of my illness in terms of "death." I had the newly acquired knowledge that I had the right and ability to fight for my own life. This does not mean that I negate all the help the medical profession gave me. I am grateful for it all. My own doctor, Dr. Paul Volberding, is a true doctor. He doctors to heal people, not just for the financial rewards. Being a medical doctor, he leans heavily on his knowledge of the medical arts. However, when I wanted to try some alternative therapy, he was very cooperative. If alternative therapy could further my healing, he was all for it. His goal and mine were the same: my complete healing.

When I got rid of the parasitical infection, my general health improved. But I was tested and retested afterward. In addition, every so often, I'm re-treated as a precaution. There is no sign of a return of the parasites or K.S. Since April of 1982, there are only a few biopsy scars; the lesions are completely gone. Some of the former lesions resemble a kind of tattoo, but they are inactive. Some have faded away totally. Actually, I had only about fourteen altogether. They were small, and all on one leg.

I did have some gamma globulin shots when I had hepatitis. I have heard Dr. Matilde Krim's theory that the gamma globulin given for hepatitis was contaminated, but I don't believe I contracted AIDS in this manner.

My belief is that the parasite is responsible for the hold AIDS got on the gay community. I recommended to my doctor that he automatically give treatment for parasites, even though he didn't find them, to his AIDS patients. Because he felt there could be side effects, he didn't like to use the treatment indiscriminately.

However, one of the people I knew was not treated for parasites. They were not found. Sometimes they are very difficult to isolate. When he wasn't treated for them, his K.S. worsened. A year later, they found the parasites, but it was too late for treatment. He died. So the time of treatment is a very important factor in healing. I feel he would be alive today if he had been given treatment automatically for his parasitical infection.

As far as drug history, I have none of any importance. In the seventies I tried everything once, but I was not a drug user and I never bought drugs myself. I haven't used any in the last ten years except in relation to medical prescriptions.

I have never had syphilis, but I had gonorrhea five times. The gay lifestyle seems to be conducive to getting gonorrhea. The passive partner in particular is susceptible. It is the passive partner who is more apt to get infected with AIDS. But with care, AIDS is not that easily given or gotten.

After my infection was under control, I had a monogamous relationship with a lover for three years. Naturally, I told him about my condition, and introduced him to Dr. Volberding. They had a private discussion about his pending relationship with me. The outcome was that he was tested for AIDS and proved to be negative. When our relationship broke up after three years, he again was tested and again proved to be negative. So my infection was not transmitted to him in spite of our close and active relationship.

Of course, I was considered cured or in remission at this time. The AIDS virus is still in my body, but I do not feel threatened by it. I feel that I can co-exist with the virus, so I don't panic. One of the important factors in my healing came from my body. Scientifically, Dr. Levi has determined that I have been manufacturing "killer" cells, suppressor cells. These cells keep out the depressor cells and are active in battling the disease. Last fall, Dr. Levi put specimens of my blood in a petri dish. When he took out the suppressor cells, the AIDS came back. When he put them back in again, the activity stopped.

Now, he's cloning these cells and storing them. Hopefully, if my body stops making them, he will have a supply to give me. He is also experimenting to see how these cells might stimulate growth of the suppressor cells in other people with this sickness. Originally, there were other individuals who were antibody positive and also had suppressor cells, but I was the only one of the group who actually had symptoms of AIDS, namely the K.S. The others who were antibody positive had not developed any symptoms.

There is a vaccine that researchers have developed and are trying out, but the suppressor cells are something different. They recognize the virus and keep it from activating. The big research question is to find out why I am producing these cells, and whether they will work for other people—or whether theirs will work for me. Each individual may have to develop his own. Also, in the study, Dr. Levi wants to discover how the body stimulates the growth of these cells, so that perhaps the stimulus could be transferred to another individual.

My system has developed a defense system of its own. Timing is important, and ridding my body of the parasitical infection gave my body time to heal itself.

In many of the early attempts to heal AIDS, it was a rush job to try to cure the patient overnight. With the venereal diseases, we're used to taking a pill or a shot and being cured in two days. I think the immune system is far more delicate and needs more time. Patience is very important. The body must have time to recognize the problem and to correct it.

The body heals itself if given the opportunity. That opportunity could be missed because the body could be clogged by treatment drugs, by several viruses attacking at once, by parasitical infections, by emotional traumas, or mental exhaustion. The body can't be overworked, overdosed, or overtreated and remain healthy.

It seems to me it's possible even to overdose on vitamins or something else that if taken properly would be beneficial. The body needs balance. But people get impatient for a cure through fear or whatever. Then they get desperate. Someone recommends herbal tea, and they wind up drinking two gallons a day. Alternative therapy is good, but you have to use common sense. You have to listen to your body and know that you're not overloading it.

I've heard hospitals criticized for taking away the patients' freedom of choice. Perhaps there are places that do this. But I don't have feelings of persecution from my hospital relationship. When I was at General, the first thing the staff did was give me the patient's bill of rights. I was always told that I had the choice of receiving chemotherapy, or whatever else the medical doctors offered.

I elected to do acupuncture twice a month as my own way of dealing with AIDS. I thought it would be a way of reducing stress and thereby improving my immune system. I was fortunate, because at this time, the hospital had its own alternative therapy clinic where they practiced acupuncture, biofeedback, aura massage, and other holistic, New Age therapies.

Aura massage was interesting and I tried it. It is a method of massage in which the masseur or masseuse does not touch the body at all. My masseuse moved her hands over my body until she came up with a visualization, which she would then work on. For instance, in going over the spinal column, she might come up with the image of a vine that's twisted, and then she would untwist the vine. Or she would go over my spleen and visualize it as an icicle. Then she would melt the icicle.

This masseuse was very sincere in what she was doing, and I think that it helped. I felt more relaxed. It was rather like the laying on of hands. I experienced aura massage only a couple of times, but I saw that it could be a good therapy for some people.

Unfortunately, since I was at the hospital, the alternative therapy wing has been discontinued. I'm not sure why, but I think the funds were limited and an existing grant was not renewed. It's too bad because I feel it was very beneficial in providing physical as well as mental relaxation, which are important to the AIDS patient in controlling stress.

In my own case, my acupuncture treatments were very helpful, and I feel they were a very important part of my healing, although I would not discount the chemotherapy or other medical treatments I received.

Acupuncture was instrumental in giving me training in relaxation, of living without stress. Once you have taken acupuncture, you can reawaken this feeling without actually having the treatment. Acupuncture is a doorway to listening to the body, of becoming conscious of the body. I feel it was beneficial in releasing the body toxins, in balancing bodily energies, and unblocking the system.

Since leaving the hospital, I have had to curtail my treatments because my insurance has stopped, and my financial situation does not allow me to continue them. I was fortunate in having long-term disability from the company I was with, and then I got social security. But my total income is only $800.00 a month. For the past five years, I've been living on that. It's not much money. I've basically been able to eat and pay the rent, but I haven't been able to buy any new clothes for five years. I would like to start acupuncture therapy again on a regular basis when I am financially able. It was good for me. Through acupuncture, it became easy for me to meditate and do creative visualization. I feel both of these therapies are beneficial to me.

It's strange, but when I was recovering from K.S., I used to visualize my cancer crumbling away like crumbling shredded wheat. Later, I saw pictures of cancer cells, and they looked just like shredded wheat.

Fear is a killer. Fear is justifiable, because so many people have died, but justification of the fear doesn't alleviate the damage it causes.

There are some people who over-react. There are people who are so horrified by the idea of having the AIDS virus in their system that they won't rest until it's totally gone, but I don't feel that way.

I feel we have all sorts of viruses and bugs in our bodies. I don't want to give the idea that one has to rid himself totally of these things. I think that what life is about is co-existence. I don't want the virus to kill me. I don't want it to get the upper hand, but at the same time, if it stays dormant in my body and doesn't give me a bad time, it can stay there. I think there's a danger in getting so paranoid that you feel you must get rid of every last bit of it. It puts a person in a high-tension position inducing the rush-to-get-well panic—which is definitely not conducive to healing, and that is what the patient really wants. We must relax and accept the fact that this alien has come into us and into our lives. I understand that emotions are strong and made stronger by the media, sometimes by the medical profession, and sometimes by talking with others. To me, the benefit of acupuncture (or other alternative therapies) is the ability to give relaxation in the face of these emotions. Visualization helps one by giving mental pictures of calmness and regeneration.

When AIDS became a recognized term, and it was

apparent that I had this infection, I had to re-establish my will to live by dealing with things one day at a time. There's always some discomfort, or something that requires a positive effort to maintain harmony and peace, but then you deal with it individually. You don't blame everything on your illness.

With hepatitis, it was easy for me to blame my liver for everything. Then I finally learned that my liver wasn't totally responsible for all my illnesses. And the same is true with the cancer, or with AIDS. It's a matter of not blaming everything on AIDS. One learns to live with AIDS. He becomes patient and awaits his healing. He must know that the body can regenerate itself; the body can fight its own fight even with something like cancer or AIDS. AIDS is many diseases, so there is not just one solution, and there is no quick cure.

I had very few symptoms with my AIDS. I did not have nausea, diarrhea, fevers or night sweats. I did periodically have thrush in my mouth, but as a whole my symptoms were not those of pain or distress. Perhaps this absence of discomfort was partially responsible for my overcoming the illness. I was able to maintain a normal mode of life in spite of it. However, I do feel that if I let myself get rundown, overloaded with work or stress, or suffer emotional imbalance or any imbalance, my immune system could be overworked and something more serious could occur.

While this is a danger hanging over my head at all times, in some ways I consider it beneficial, because it is the leash that keeps my activities in check. As my lifestyle has always been a basically healthful one, this discipline is not difficult to maintain, but the situation adds an incentive to continue to maintain it and not get lax.

There's an awareness that you develop in terms of what you can do. It's a specific consciousness in terms of physical, mental and spiritual relationships. You cannot exist for very long when you are at war with yourself. In terms of stress, I have come to realize that living in the present is very important as opposed to getting caught up with the past or future. Living in the moment is important. To abstract the meaning of that moment, one must let fears, frustration, anger and in fact all inharmonies flow away, leaving you with the moment and peace.

Some people become reclusive. They believe everything negative they hear, and they withdraw. They block everything. They don't allow themselves to heal. There's no way under these conditions they can process the disease out of themselves. You do have to wage psychological warfare. You have to learn how to think positively. You have to be in control. You can't let the disease control you!

I find that expression of feelings is very helpful to relieve built-up tensions or stress. Whatever your feelings or emotions are, if you get them out in the open, it's easier to get rid of them, or at least they will lessen. It's a way of eliminating the toxins from your body. The Chinese believe you can eliminate toxins not only by diet, but by self-expression and creativity. If you have a hobby, an art form, something you can bury yourself in, and be surrounded by pleasant thoughts, this can help eliminate toxins.

But some people can't talk about it, and can't express it. They're afraid, not only of AIDS, but of the whole gay picture. These are the people who must learn to love themselves, to develop self-esteem and to cherish it. It can be a healer.

The community I live in has helped me a great deal. I feel fortunate to live in San Francisco in its gay community. There is a support system here, and I can channel into it. But again, you have to be wary of channeling into a support system which is teaching one how to die. There are people who do not like Shanti. (The Shanti Project deals with emotional and practical support for Persons With AIDS and their families.) They feel it is teaching PWAs to die "properly." You should be seeking to live, not die. I don't believe everyone has this opinion about Shanti, but getting into a death trip is a danger. Fear mushrooms, and as it grows, it becomes proportionately difficult or impossible to control. I can't actually say much about Shanti, because I haven't really participated in it. My conviction is that definitely, they should be teaching one to live with AIDS, to overcome it, as opposed to dying with it.

I have not had much to do with Louise Hay or other support groups because of the way I was diagnosed. By the time I had AIDS, I had already worked out my approach to the cure for K.S., and being a basic approach to health, it was what I needed to control AIDS. In effect, I was well on the way to recovery before I knew I was sick.

Gay men are susceptible for many reasons, one of which is the idea of being a disgrace to society, which sits in judgment. It has cast the gay man off—treated him like a second class citizen, with the result that he falls prey to his own low self-esteem.

The Federal government seemed to be unconcerned about AIDS when it was attacking the gays, the drug users and the prostitutes, but now that AIDS is getting out into the general population, it is becoming concerned. But we, the gays, are a part of the general population, just as much as any other group. The government or the "straight" population seems to want to make a dichotomy between the "good" guys and the "bad." The whole red herring of the mandatory testing is another way of isolating us as a group. They don't deal with the reality of the situation by increasing sex education in schools, or supplying condoms. They're trying to isolate the disease by testing people and coming up with lists. To them, that makes more political sense—and a more organized and efficient approach to a possible cure.

Sex education is important in helping to control the disease. When Dr. Volberding talked with my lover before we started our relationship, he recommended the use of condoms. I consider that the safe sex we had for three years was directly attributable to the use of condoms. I have heard of cases where one of two lovers did go out with another, who unknown to him, had AIDS. The person was basically monogamous, but became infected without knowing it, and subsequently infected his partner. They both wound up dying—from a single exposure. From my own personal experience, I would say this is rare if safe sex procedures are followed. I have also heard of cases where the diagnoses have proved to be incorrect. Again, I have heard of people who were diagnosed as having AIDS who committed suicide. Being human, we are all subject to error, but when the diagnosis of AIDS is given, there should be understanding and counseling given with it. This is a traumatic time for the individual, and he should not be left to the mercy of his overactive imagination.

Fear and the desire to know whether they are free of the virus has driven many people to take the test for AIDS. Maybe two or three years ago, they were involved with someone who they now discover has AIDS. These tests gross $6,500,000,000 (billion dollars) or more a year, which is big business, and big business is sometimes not interested in the individual.

When a friend becomes infected with AIDS, one feels helpless. He's filled with grief and deep emotions, which have to be faced and balanced. Many of my long-time friends have died. I've made new ones, but you don't make friends overnight, not like those you've known for so long. My film-maker friend died in New York. I wrote music for him which was in one of his films. I had known him since 1973. Another friend who died was the musical director of two of my shows. The second show was the one I was writing when I was first diagnosed as having AIDS. He helped me score the music, and each week we worked on another song. He was very supportive of me during the period of my initial diagnosis.

The first people to acquire AIDS suffered the greatest number of fatalities, because so little was known about AIDS. It was believed to affect only the gay community. It was called "The Gay Plague," and there was a certain indifference to it by the entire country.

I had a friend whose lover had died the year before. He had been living with AIDS for some time, but with the loss of his lover, he went steadily downhill. There was nothing anyone could do to help. A year later, on the anniversary of his lover's death, he died. This reveals the power of the subconscious, and that there is a will to live, and a will to die.

There was another case of a friend who had successfully fought AIDS off for years. He would respond negatively to it and go downhill, then he would bounce back to apparent good health. This went on for several years; then he suddenly started downhill again, and didn't recover. These are the cases that make one realize there is much to know not only about AIDS, but about those who have it—about people, and the power of the mind.

I feel strongly, of course, that my one friend died of emotional causes totally distinct from his virus infection, but the other one—what would suddenly cause him to backslide? Was it emotional? Was he just tired of fighting? Or was there a physical cause like losing the ability to manufacture his depressor cells? These are questions that need answers, and doubtless we will get the answers in the future.

AIDS has affected my life in ways other than losing my friends. It caused me to lose my job, but my employment was not that exciting and in losing it, I actually found new doors opening. I became totally involved in volunteering to share my experience, and this resulted in public appearances. I was one of the founding members of the San Francisco AIDS Foundation and was on its board for three years, through 1986. I was also on the AIDS Action Council Board. I was the first person with AIDS on that board, which has a national lobby in Washington, D.C. I helped set up the San Francisco People With AIDS group. So, I was very active in volunteering in AIDS work. I did public speaking at health forums, appeared on local and national TV, (Channels 5, 7, and 2), and other local media.

I was recently interviewed by the *Los Angeles Times*. So this illness was, I feel, really a blessing.

Certainly, there have been 25,000 deaths, but how many have lived? That's basically why I have done these interviews—to let people know that life is possible after AIDS. It's obviously a very serious situation. I'd like the media to investigate the Federal government to find out why it has been dragging its heels in coping with the AIDS crisis.

The San Francisco General Hospital has a model outpatient system. The whole structure is set up in an efficient manner, and it has been successful. Very few people go to the hospital until near the very end. The whole approach here has been one to save money for the people. They have support groups, and the patient doesn't have to deal with expensive hospitalization for long periods. The staff must deal with the hysteria of people occasionally. Some people are very nervous about touching, being around, or even seeing persons with AIDS. For instance, I was talking with a man one time, and some saliva flew off my lip and hit his. He was petrified that he was going to get AIDS. This was a very uncomfortable situation for both of us. Now people know more about it, and they realize it's not that easy to catch AIDS.

I believe that sexual activity is a part of normal life. I believe in safe sex, as proved from my own experience. Although I was the passive partner, I feel the fact that my lover used a condom kept the relationship from being a threatening one to him. We had sexual intercourse for two years before breaking up. He was still free of infection at that time.

For the past two years, I've been dating. Safe sex is possible, and the condom, properly used, will provide it. If you don't feel safe with one, use two. If there is a really large ejaculation and leakage, infection may be possible. The passive partner is usually the one to be infected, but it can happen either way. I go both ways. In the last two years, I've been primarily active. I think that the primary method of transmission is anally—in terms of sex. I periodically had anal bleeding. There would be abrasions or something that caused bleeding. The rectum is a vulnerable area.

It doesn't seem as if infection would be a problem with oral sex. I've never been into that. Many AIDS patients have thrush or sores in their mouth. If that's the case, I believe the partners should seek professional advice on how to keep their relationship on a safe level.

I do believe in safe sex. Sex is important. People are not going to give it up. However, one doesn't have to have intercourse every time one has sex. The partners can mutually masturbate and do a few things that are pleasurable without having intercourse. Also, I would recommend not having intercourse unless the other person is a consistent partner. I would only want to have mutual masturbation, or something else that I know would be extremely safe.

Most of the time, I tell the person about my health condition, but sometimes I haven't done so. That's when I knew we were only going to masturbate. If there's going to be any kind of kissing or intercourse, I want them to know. I feel it's their prerogative to make the choice about the outcome.

The changes AIDS has brought into my life have all been positive. Immediately after going on disability, I became involved in writing a musical show. That was a source of liberation. Since I was diagnosed with AIDS, I've written two musical shows, both of which have been produced. One ran six weeks, and one was done in the workshop at the California State University at Berkeley.

Although I lost my job because of AIDS, it has helped me with my life and career. I am back at school now studying for my master's degree in social work. I've completed two years, and this fall, hopefully, I'll finish all the requirements.

I applied for a grant to help me financially. I got almost all the required paper work in. It is very complicated, but I stayed with it until I was asked to send in financial statements from all the schools I've attended. That involved four different schools and a lot of time. I gave up. I was right in the middle of writing a play for a festival. I already have a master's degree in fine arts and playwriting.

I do want to continue my work in the arts, but my new field will give me more job options. Hopefully, I can become employed and get job benefits, because, when I go back to work, I'll lose social security and the long-term benefits from my former employer.

I would like to do counseling. That's my goal, but I also want to write and compose music. Since getting AIDS, I have become more involved in medical and social work, but I consider my career to be in the arts.

However, as previously mentioned, since this illness has entered my life, I have become more involved with the general public, in the media, on panel forums, and with interviews.

The media in their questioning had a tendency to ask, rather sensationally or dramatically, "How does it feel to know you'll be dead in two months?" That was in the beginning stages. They would play up the mortality of the illness. Now, within the last two years, I get more people calling me to do stories of survival. Many people desire to know whether I can point to one treatment principle for a cure, but I cannot. Some want to hear that alternative therapy is the sole answer—I assume because they have lost faith in traditional medicine and its 100% fatality rate. But there is no one treatment, no one cure. I believe in alternative therapies, but not over traditional medical procedures. The cure is the harmonious combination of things that are specific to each individual. It's a whole new way of listening to your body and knowing your own life. You have to make decisions and choices all through life. These decisions must not result in stress or an overload on the immune system. It's a common sense thing, in terms of eating well, exercising, resting. All those things continue to apply—

and to everyone.

I do feel that natural food is the best food. I'm not on a strictly macrobiotic diet, but I know that grains are important. I've always eaten a lot of grains, long before my illness. Grains, fresh vegetables and fruit are important in the diet. I don't eat much red meat. I do consume dairy products. One should use common sense: three meals a day of good food—no junk foods. I rarely eat candy, but if you're eating well, I don't think it hurts to eat sweets on occasion.

I know people who have been on government assistance with a limited amount of money coming in each week. They spend it on movies and popcorn, not on a good diet. There are people whose bodies are rundown, because they just don't have enough money for food, and what little they have is not spent wisely.

You should use every resource you have. My religious background is Christian, so I feel I have Christian resources to help me. I think the power of prayer and the healing possible with spiritual imagery is strong. I have always had what I consider a spiritual contact. If the treatment is meaningful to you, use it!

I definitely do not believe that the gay person or the gay community is being punished by God. If you love yourself in the right perspective to the rest of the world, you automatically know that God is a Being of unlimited, divine Love—and you are loved.

The primary change in my sexual practices since AIDS has been in the use of a condom. However, the longest relationship I ever had was after I discovered my infection. Also, I have had more affairs that last several months, not just for one occasion. Before AIDS, I was probably having three different partners every week. So there is a change in my sex pattern, from numerous individuals to consistent partners.

It's easier to tell someone about your health situation in the quiet of your own home, so when occasionally I date someone new—if the person is interested enough to come to my place or for me to go to his, prior to intercourse, I tell him the whole story.

On the whole, I think this disease has made us all more responsible in regard to each other's bodies. We realize now that we have to treat our bodies with respect in terms of our health. Earlier, sex was considered a liberating thing. I don't regret my sexual exploration during the seventies, but at the same time, now I know that gonorrhea, syphilis, hepatitis, parasitical infections, and AIDS are realities that have to be dealt with. We are learning how to deal with them.

I have never negated the good I have received from the medical profession and traditional medicine.

In the sunny Mission area of San Francisco, there is a many-storied building with sprawling wings that offered me shelter from the storms of my panic.

My sincere hope is that those who are anxious about their condition, those who wonder if they have been infected with AIDS, will go to a qualified medical center for testing. My deep prayer is that they will find one, as I did, that is without prejudice—one that will be involved in caring for their health, and one that will offer them immediately, when they first enter, the patient's bill of rights.

WHAT DANIEL TURNER DID

• He had support from his doctor who was involved, caring and receptive, who put the care of his patients first. His doctor allowed Daniel to choose other healing modalities.

• He took care of himself by slowing down and becoming more self-reliant.

• He felt the benefits of acupunture and aura massage.

• He was determined to wage a war on AIDS and fight to win.

• He believed that parasites were responsible for his sickness.

• He did not panic. He felt that if the AIDS virus was in his body, he could co-exist with it.

• He felt that healing is not a rush job; the body must have plenty of time to recognize the problem and correct it.

• He let fear, frustration, anger, and all inharmonies dissolve in love.

• He understood that emotional problems often develop into physical problems.

• His self-expression and creativity were developed.

• He stayed away from organizations that teach how to "die properly."

• He believes that if a treatment is meaningful to you, it should be used.

• He knows that the cure for AIDS is a harmonious combination of many health-producing measures that are specific to each individual.

• Daniel Turner sought to live and not to die. He is now "alive and well."

Tommy Griggs

Tommy Griggs is a slender, intense and intelligent young man who has a rare sense of humor. He has that beautiful quality of being able to laugh easily. Tommy was diagnosed as having pneumocystis pneumonia in April of 1987.

Tommy Griggs' Adventure

The best place to start is the beginning of my life, because I believe that my illness, in part, begins that far back. I was born in Fresno, California. I was an only child and grew up with my mother and stepfather. My mother's influence was the greater in my life. She was one of ten children and had a difficult time growing up. She brought some of her problems to her marriage, and to her role as mother.

My natural father kidnapped me when I was three or four years old and took me to another state. My mother came after me and brought me home. I was never given an explanation as to why the adults were behaving as they were. I believe I absorbed some of the feelings of anxiety in my family, and not having another explanation, I believe I blamed myself. It's possible that this was the beginning of my inability to love myself.

My folks provided well for me in all the material ways. I was not abused or neglected physically, but they could not give me emotional support. There were no hugs; there was never a sign of affection; there were few reassurances. I couldn't talk to anyone about my feelings.

The atmosphere in our home was totally negative. Still, I know my family loves me and would do anything they can to help me. The problem was that I had begun to hate or at least dislike myself. My folks were not church-going people, but they had a "Christian belief," and I was very much affected by that. The only church I knew was on television, and I didn't want any part of what to me were hate mongers. So I grew up without any sense of God. I think that lack of affection is one of the illnesses of our generation. All my life I have craved affection. Affection is very healing for me, and I am sure, for everyone.

In school I felt myself to be the "nerd"; I have always been self-conscious. When I was entering school life, I needed someone to show me how to play ball and join in athletics. I felt I had some potential and if given a chance, I would have done fairly well, but I was shy and not aggressive, and no one showed me how to play. So I didn't learn to join in sports, and this fact isolated me further from my peers.

I thought I was too thin, and I was confused about what a person is supposed to be in this world. The negative atmosphere in my home contributed to my lack of confidence. Since there was no emotional support, I floundered and struggled on without the inner confidence it takes to be happy and fulfilled. Along with a negative sense of myself, I had to deal with my own strong emotions.

My need to be loved has taken me down many paths in life. My lifestyle caused me to become more sophisticated about the world than the others in my family. I have come to certain understandings they are not aware of nor would they share. I had no time for thoughts of success because simply trying to function had to take second place to my need to deal with powerful emotions. As I grew older, I moved around a great deal. I worked as a waiter, was a good one, and kept moving. I lived in Texas, Arizona, California, and Hawaii. I usually stayed in a place for about six months, and then moved on. I paid no attention to my diet or my health. I usually have a healthy appetite, and I suppose I'm thin for some other reason than poor appetite. I was very promiscuous, but I seldom allowed anyone to love me. I frequented the bathhouses. I found some measure of good feelings from just being held; the physical contact with another body allowed me to feel alive and distracted me enough so I didn't have to deal with my suffering spirit. I think most people suffer from excessive lust at times, some more than others. The sexual encounters distracted me from the real problem. The difference now is that affection is very important to me.

While I lived in Los Angeles in 1977, I had occasion to talk to a lady who had been to see a psychic. She raved about this man and his talents. For some reason I was interested, but angry at myself for being so. I was sure it was "hogwash," yet I went to see the man, ostensibly to be able to say he was a fake. But he wasn't; he performed a healing for me at that time, and I did not know it. He brought out so much old stuff that had needed uncovering for so long.

Then he taught me a technique for meditation. He told me that I had many strengths, and there was a new path for me to take. I started moving in circles with people who meditate.

This started me thinking beyond my limited lifestyle, based on physical sensation. Meditation became a part of me, and worked for me in visible ways. Later, I found out how deeply it will work if you are able to allow it. I noticed there was no organization set up for gay people to learn to meditate. More than many others, we need the healing effects of metaphysical studies. I had taken part in workshops, and had been a student of meditation, but I had never led a group. I felt I knew so little about meditation, but perhaps what I knew could help others. A voice inside me began telling me: "start a group." My usual lack of confidence caused me to hesitate: I wasn't learned enough in the field; I had never led a meditation group; there was no one else I could turn to for help. But the inner voice persisted and became more demanding until I started a group. So the Gay Metaphysical-Spiritual Association (G.M.S.A.) came into being.

That was seven years ago, and the organization is now functioning nationwide. I started a branch in Long Beach, California. The G.M.S.A has given me the best of all gifts—the ability to share. Now I know what I want to do, and how I want to live.

I was flowering into the great potential of the person I could become. What a person can do or be is infinite. At G.M.S.A., we teach self-love and have a grand time doing it.

There was a conflict between what meditation was teaching me and my lifestyle. The conflict was in the giving and receiving of love. I didn't know it at the time; I thought I was just depressed. Treating my body abusively was a burden to it. I went into business with a friend who is now my partner. We had a good product, and wanted to manufacture and sell it. We were starting the business on a shoestring and the bills were coming in; we were struggling.

About this time, I got syphilis and gonorrhea. I was given antibiotics in each case. I struggled on, and so did my immune system. I seldom drink alcohol, I don't smoke, I don't use recreational drugs, but I have taken a lot of antibiotics.

For business reasons, I made a trip to Mexico. There I drank some polluted water. I think my illness really came full circle at this time. Something else could have caused it, but I think the water was responsible for my amoebiasis. I was very sick.

I returned home and went to a doctor who "antibiot-icked" me almost to death. Even then I didn't wait to see the thing healed. The business needed me; I went back to work, but I was very depressed. It was getting worse. When the lungs are affected the patient gets feelings of depression, according to principles of Chinese medicine. I was diagnosed as depressed and given an anti-depressant drug. I accepted the diagnosis of depression; my lungs were collapsing as I lay there at home. That drug nearly killed me. I had no money, so I didn't try to get medical attention. I believed the rumors that if you have no money, you can't see a doctor. So my condition went untreated. Finally, I collapsed.

From this point on, it is hearsay for awhile, because during this time I was unconscious. I found out later that my mother, cousin and aunt came from Fresno to get me. They took me to a hospital that trains interns, but we were turned away. Then we went to the Bennett Clinic in Long Beach, California. This is a wonderful place, a private clinic. They took me in without money. I was tested for pneumocystis pneumonia and the results were positive. The first thing they did was get oxygen into me and then IVs. As soon as they got a bed in ICU, they intubated me with the respirator. They told my family that it would not breathe for me, but would help me breathe. I was on the respirator for about a week, and then I awakened. All I could think was "where am I?" and "what have these people done to me?" It's strange to wake up with all those tubes in you. I didn't know that I had almost died. Emergency medicine saved my life.

It's very important to realize that whether or not you

have money, you can get medical attention. The Bennett Clinic was very good to me. They knew I was gay and had AIDS, but did not treat me like a leper. They helped me, although I had no money.

After I was released, Dr. Ron Loya of the Bennett Clinic became my doctor. He has patients who are listening to the teachings of Louise Hay, and believes there are other things besides drugs that work. He is interested in holistic healing, and is very open minded. It is good to have a doctor who is not totally clinical and can encompass other ways of healing besides drugs.

I was moved to Harbor General Hospital, UCLA. Harbor is a county hospital, but they took good care of me. The nurses and assistants knew I had AIDS, they knew how close I was to death, but they made me laugh about something every day. They are overworked and underpaid; I wonder why and how they do it. I was in the hospital for total bedrest for thirty days. The fact that I didn't die gave me a positive path to take, and I didn't even think of death after that. I knew I was still alive for some reason. The opinion was that I had a terminal disease, but I could find a positive thought for every negative reason anyone could give me. I felt very sick, but inside I was healing.

Harbor General Hospital of UCLA is a good hospital, and the people who work there do not treat you like a leper; they are kind and professional. If you are in need of medical treatment, you should get to a doctor any way you can. If I had gotten medical treatment sooner, I might not have had to go through a brush with death, and all the fear and weakness that it produces. The people at Harbor General Hospital are very informed concerning AIDS, and I'm sure there are other hospitals around the country where people can get good treatment. After all, since AIDS isn't a gay disease, the public will have to deal with it. The doctors are practicing on us with experimental programs. We are in the forefront of this battle.

When I was tested for AIDS, they started out with the ELISA test. If that is positive, they do the Western Blot test. These are the two blood tests. If both are positive, they say it is conclusive—the person has AIDS. But AIDS is based on signs and symptoms. There are people who get a positive result in both tests and do not have AIDS. That is called a false positive. There are false negatives, too. So, the tests are very controversial, because they are not totally reliable.

While in the hospital, I was not allowed to move around. My doctor was Dr. Lynne Chang. She was wonderful—very positive, and she cared. It showed. She got me started on the positive path, and it was up to me to keep that positive state of mind. The nurses and health-care workers were excellent. When they finally took all the tubes out of me, I was already in a very positive state of mind. And the mind is crucial in healing.

I have thought a great deal about how I came to get AIDS. It's true there is a virus, but I think the damage to the immune system starts long before the virus manifests. The virus is transmitted sexually, that is clear. In that sense, it could be considered another venereal disease. But IV drug users and people who receive blood transfusions also get the virus. Since almost anyone can become infected by this disease, AIDS has stimulated much research.

My mother came to stay with me for three weeks a while ago. We are very close now, and she has made me understand how much she loves me. I love her, but she has accepted the media's abundant negativity and does not have faith in my recovery. It makes me angry that she won't believe in my recovery, but in another way, I understand it and feel sorry for her.

Let's face it. If you are homosexual, and you have AIDS, you are a social outcast. But I am fortunate. I have never been treated like an abomination. I hear the stories of people being forced to leave their homes; people who are burned out because they have AIDS (even children!); people who aren't allowed to work or go to school. I am sad about this, but it has not happened to me. My business partner and I were working hard, and suddenly I was disabled. He has carried on the business and is doing well. He has been a great help to me throughout and I hope to be able to return to work before long, so I consider myself lucky. I don't like to say this, but it seems that people in small southern towns are the most violent against gays. I was raised in that kind of atmosphere. And these ignorant, violent people claim to be "good Christians."

I came home from the hospital. My friends had found Ed who helped me every day while I stayed in my apartment in Long Beach. I couldn't have pulled through it without him. Ed is in an excellent state program to help those on state aid. California pays half his salary, and the person being helped pays the other half. A wonderful friend pitched in and paid my half. Ed did my laundry and cooked for me. He drove me around in my car to buy groceries, pay bills, and do all of the draining things that limit one's life's energy.

At one point (six months to a year before getting sick), I was given Erythromycin, an antibiotic, for a dental infection which was causing fevers. The drug gave me awful cramps. I had a terrible reaction. This dental infection has remained a problem since coming home.

I believe I was immuno-suppressed before I got the symptoms of AIDS—at least three years before. When doctors keep giving people vaccines and antibiotics, it suppresses the immune system, and that's what happened to me. It doesn't happen all at once, but takes a while to manifest. Junk foods, fast foods, and antibiotics are factors that weaken the body. The neglected latchkey children are the new generation of weak people especially at risk. Looking back at it now, I can see a decline in my energy level. The last time I really felt good was about three years before the onset of AIDS.

When I was first diagnosed, I didn't know anyone with AIDS. I did not have a friend who had died or anything like that. I was the first Person With AIDS I had ever met! Later, I met people at the PWA (People With AIDS) groups. There is a camaraderie there; everyone knows that all the others have it. We are able to sympathize with each other and exchange important information.

The people who are using the drug AZT have to take the drug every four hours, twenty-four hours a day. Each one can identify with the problems of people on AZT. Waking up every four hours to take a pill is no fun. Everybody has his pill box at the meetings. Some can laugh at themselves, and that is very healing. It was difficult for me in these groups, because I have never been a person who was able to enter a group and function well. I don't present myself well, but somewhat stay off in a corner. My shyness was painful, and it kept me away from social groups. Although I did make friends, it took me some time because of my reserve. This problem didn't occur for me while leading a group in meditation. With my meditation groups, I felt more in charge of myself. I believe that shyness is really a lack of self-esteem. If that is so, no wonder it is so painful.

I saw Dr. Ron Loya at the Bennett Medical Center every two weeks. He was comfortable with my spiritual endeavors. When my last T-cell reading was low, he suggested that I focus on my meditation.

One day, in the meditation room of a teacher, I saw a picture of the face of Sai Baba, the Indian spiritual master, and something happened to me. I could not go on with the class until she told me who he was. She gave me a book about him which I still have. I am not much of a reader, but I worked my way through two of his books. It was wonderful to discover that there is someone out there who believes in the power of tenderness. I have never seen Sai Baba in person, and I do not write him or talk to him. But as I understand it, what he does as a Master is affect the inner person. He can come to you spiritually, if you need him; he has a profound effect on your inner feelings. It is strange, and most people won't believe it, but it is a happening in the Universal Consciousness.

I am aware of the strong connection between the food we eat and the state of our health. I eat chicken, fish, lots of fruits, vegetables, grains and nuts, and stay away from all red meat. I like Mexican food, and I feel that it is quite healthful.

I tried to be a vegetarian for a while but realized that I don't know enough about food and food combinations to remain healthy under this discipline. I plan on looking into all the alternative methods of healing that have come to my attention.

Concerning "safe sex": condoms inhibit the transfer of bodily fluids, and early withdrawals also help protect partners. I don't care for the idea of celibacy. I have heard of tantra yoga as a method for sublimating the sex drive, but I don't know anything about it, and I don't know anyone who does.

I know that I find affection a most satisfying expression of real love. How to deal with lust is the problem I have. Perhaps if we all could open ourselves more to love expressed through affection, we could find a healthy satisfaction there.

I have never enjoyed the passive position in a sex relationship. An intelligent approach to sex, would be to always use a condom, have an affectionate partner, don't go to bars where people get so absolutely stoned they don't know what is going on. Don't pick up just anybody and take him home with you. Recognize your low self-esteem problem and begin to affirm that you are God's child. You have a right to be here.

Begin to do things that make you feel good about yourself. Try to heal the wound of no self-esteem. Begin to care about yourself so that you consider what you eat and care whether or not you sleep, what kind of drugs you use and what kind of toxins you take into your body and your mind. Be alert. Protect yourself.

I have prayed very much during my illness, but when I pray, I do not beg and plead with God for my life. I affirm my health. I express my love and my thankfulness for another day of life. I am grateful for all the help I received.

When I thought I would die, I came up with the usual regrets: "I wish I had," "If only I had," etc., but I did not linger in that space.

When one is ill, the process of recovery is slow and difficult. The best way to help yourself is to make sure there is laughter at least once a day. Laughter is very healing. I understand that Roger Walther (one of those interviewed for this book), is writing a book on laughter therapy.

My deepest emotions have been opened. I become teary-eyed often. I savor every moment of life. I feel rushes of tenderness. I am so much more sensitive to everything. I know I will not become "thick-skinned" again, because I meditate. That's a way of life for me now.

I believe that the virus is still with me. After all, my immune system was trashed. I am working on my thought patterns and my belief system, trying to become more dedicated to my higher self. This is a difficult but exciting task.

I believe that one can continue to be re-exposed to AIDS. Many medical people feel that AIDS is one disease that comes about by continual re-exposure. One of the things people seem to be ignoring or missing is the fact that you can keep getting re-infected.

When I think of my future—which isn't often since I am concerned with the present—I recognize the need to make money and deal with all the practical aspects of life. But there is something else now. Within the structure of the G.M.S.A., I have seen wonderful healings take place, healings of the spirit. I have seen young men come to our group barely able to overcome their own pain long enough to hide in the corner of the room. It takes some time, but before too long the same young men begin to flower, begin to understand that they are worthwhile and beautiful people whom God loves. We support each other in our efforts to live as gay men and not kill ourselves in the process. I have made wonderful friends in this way. I would like to do spiritual work in the future. Whatever form it takes, however, it is up to a Power greater than I. But that is what I would like to do. Serve the people, my people, and in that way , all of this pain and suffering that I have gone through will become a positive force in my life.

I don't feel pity for those who die, whether they are young or old. I don't want anyone to feel pity for me when I die. It's just what happens in this life. The body dies, but the spirit is eternal. Perhaps I was given the task of this illness so that I could pass on what I have learned to others, to help them overcome. Helping others is what is really important.

The best thing I could tell another person is: LIVE— whether you get the virus or not—LIVE. Take each day and make it into a day where you give and receive love. Do something to make yourself feel better every day. Enjoy the brief time we have here. Learn to live for today. If there is something negative in your life, get away from it to something positive. Be affectionate and enjoy the healing aspects of affection. Keep reaching for a better state of health, physically, spiritually and mentally. On all levels—reach for your own life and live it as you see fit.

* * * * *

It is one year later.

I have moved to Fresno (California) to live with my parents so that I can continue making my car payments.

Since being here I have lectured to four groups on "A Positive Approach to AIDS." I'm also leading a holistic support group called "Being Alive". A fairly long article about me appeared in the *Fresno Bee*.

The Church of Religious Science has been a tremendous help in my healing. The people are very loving and the teachings ring so true.

In October of 1987, I had a healer named Gene Egedio work on me. Twenty years of inner "garbage" was cleaned out in two days. He has been working with many terminally ill people with great success.

WHAT TOMMY GRIGGS DID

• He went to a private clinic, where his doctor co-operated with his desire to have alternative, natural therapies. At the clinic, the attitudes of the staff were healing for him. Humor, hope, and positive healing words were dispensed, rather than negativity and prognosis of death.

• He realized that the testing for AIDS is controversial and sometimes inaccurate, so he did not put much credence in the results.

• He studied natural therapies and holistic methods of healing that came to his attention.

• He realized how important a positive state of mind is.

• He knew that the healing powers are within oneself, but outside influences can help also— positive persons, books, natural therapies, etc.

• He used new knowledge of factors such as nutrition, supplements, etc.

- He changed his diet from "junk" foods to a nourishing, healthful nutritional plan.

- He was sympathetic toward others who also had the disease, and shared his positive attitudes and his path to recovery.

- He was alert to the harm of negative influences, and protected himself against them.

- During his illness, he prayed often and made many positive affirmations.

- He realized that laughter and expressing one's emotions are important in healing.

- He learned to love himself unconditionally.

- He overcame his shyness and lack of self-confidence, the result of a negative home atmosphere during childhood, and his consequent sense of isolation and self-condemnation.

- He learned to express his need to love himself and others in better ways.

- He realized that the physical contact that he so deeply needed could not be nourished by lust and that his suffering spirit could not be quelled with promiscuity.

- He began to unravel his false self-image and build a higher self-image.

• He taught himself techniques of meditation. He started to move in circles where people meditated, and this helped to change his environment and lifestyle.

• He found that meditation became an important part of his life; that practice had a power that was expressed outwardly in visible ways in his life.

• Feeling that others had similar needs to his, he started gay meditation groups, first in Texas, then in Long Beach, California, and Fresno, California.

• He developed a clear definition of what he wanted to do and how he wanted to live his life.

• Tommy Griggs today looks forward to a long, happy, and purposeful life, that will continue to be a blessing to himself and others.

MEDITATION

A number of the Conquerors used meditation in their holistic healing programs. There are many forms of meditation and many places where one can get training. Here is one:

The Himalayan International Institute of Yoga Science and Philosophy, R. R. 1, Box 400, Honesdale, PA 18431 (717/253-5551)

It is a nonprofit organization dedicated to teaching the various aspects of yoga and meditation as a means to foster the personal growth of the individual and the betterment of society. The Institute conducts numerous educational, therapeutic and research programs. Its Quarterly gives a guide to programs and other offerings.

This brief analysis of meditation is reprinted from the Himalayan Institute Quarterly (Spring 1988 issue):

Meditation is the uninterrupted flow of the mind towards one object or concept, and with this flow intuitive knowledge dawns. All methods of yoga prepare one to reach the state of meditation, for only through meditation can one reach the level of the superconscious mind and hence attain perfection.

Why is meditation necessary? Just as there is a subconscious state beneath the conscious state, so is there a superconscious state above the conscious state. Meditation alone can take man to this blissful state of the mind....

Meditation can also help one to overcome physical and psychological problems. A large percentage of all diseases are psychosomatic, arising from conflicts, repressions and suppressions in the unconscious mind. Meditation leads one to an awareness of these conflicts and helps one to analyze them and then erase them, thus establishing harmony at the unconscious level.

—Sri Swami Rama, *Lectures on Yoga* (Founder of Institute)

MEDITATION AND MENTALPHYSICS

In the Science of Mentalphysics, Meditation becomes less a science of the mind than a definite and conscious uncovering of the Eternal Creative Spirit of Life within ourselves. All true seekers of wisdom recognize that entering the silence is a vital way, a holy secret, for Meditation consciously links us to God and ushers us into understanding of all that is God-given.

As philosophers, we recognize also that Meditation is the final connecting link between the *outer* and *inner* man. When we regularly meditate, cultivating the inner life, the environment of the world will not master us. In Meditation we transcend thoughts, fears, actions, judgements and modes of life rather than fall into the moulds of the *race mind* . A higher wisdom catches us and transforms us into a divine pattern that enables us to express our fuller potential, overcome challenges and express the divine perfection that is our birthright as children of our creator.

There are numerous ways to go into Meditation and the right way for one is not always right for another...but as we seek, we find. Mentalphysics offers various methods which have proven successful for most seekers. Regardless of the method, regular practice daily—preferably at the same time and in the same place—enhances one's progress.

A practical, provable formula is offered for victorious living, self-mastery and a fuller expression of the gift of life.

For further information:
MENTALPHYSICS, P.O. Box 640, Yucca Valley, CA 92286-0640, Phone (619) 365-8371.

Douglas Johnson

Clarence Douglas Johnson III dotes on his eleven nieces and nephews, who range in age from less than one year to 22 years. Only 29 himself when he was diagnosed as having Kaposi's sarcoma, his first thoughts were of them, of all the lifetimes he would miss—their precious lives as they evolved. If he died—and wasn't AIDS a death sentence? —he would miss it all.

Douglas Johnson's Adventure

When I heard the biopsy results, I kept thinking, "Oh God, I don't want to die. I don't want to die." In my mind's eye, I was seeing my youngest nephew. He was just six months old then, and I wanted to watch him grow up. It was unbearable to think I'd be cut off, unable to enjoy this newest gift of life to our family.

I'm very close to my nephews and nieces; I'm like a second father to them. They always spend Christmas and vacations with me, and I've watched all of them growing up. I love them all; I'm involved in their lives, and I thought, what a loss! Not to be able to see them develop —my sisters' children. I felt there was so much more I wanted to do, but that I was going to be cheated out of it by this certain and early death.

Then, in the middle of all this turmoil, I realized that I was going to be cheated as much as I wanted to be—that I had a choice whether I was to live or die. And I decided that I didn't have to die. Whatever it would take, psychologically or physically, I knew I had to educate myself to do it. I had a road ahead of me—maybe rough, but a road, a learning experience. And it has been quite a learning experience.

That first day, though, and for almost the next two weeks, the thought that I was going to die would keep popping into my head. I thought I'd be O.K., but then I'd get depressed and start thinking about dying, and I'd go on a crying jag. I did that until I couldn't cry any more.

When I was diagnosed, the treatment recommended to me was AZT, but I refused it. I thought there might be side effects outweighing any possible value. Anyway, I said no. It didn't sound right to me.

My friends were shocked by the news, but their shock quickly turned into concern. My family was very worried, and very supportive. What really helped me was the arrival of my sister. She came down from San Francisco within five days of my telling her, even though her baby was only six months old and was being breast-fed. She arrived and was ready to go— to clinics, doctors, nutritionists—to look into every possible alternative.

I had already learned a little about the holistic approach and, as far as I was concerned, it was the only way to go. The holistic and spiritual—the combination worked for me.

My sister called at least two or three times a week after returning home. She's about eight years older, and we've always been close. She's a very positive person and always has been. She's the one who helped me most in my recovery.

The doctors were supportive also. I made the decision, based on my research and, I suppose, my own sense of what I needed. The nutritionist later told me he was very impressed with my attitude.

I was encouraged by books I read, such as *Conquering AIDS Now!*, (Gregory and Leonardo) and many Church of Religious Science books. One of these in particular, called *New Design for Living* by Dr. Ernest Holmes, is a wonderful book I'd recommend to anyone. *This Thing Called You* and *This Thing Called Life* are two books by Holmes that changed my life. I learned to change my thoughts and beliefs; this helped me with the AIDS diagnosis. I really didn't ever flip out over it.

Another work that inspired me was *Love, Medicine and Miracles*, by Bernie S. Siegel, M.D. He's a surgeon at Yale who works with cancer patients. He calls them "exceptional patients." They all were diagnosed as having "terminal" cancer, but he worked with them, and they pulled through, because they learned they could heal themselves. So, their healing started from within and, no matter how much cobalt or chemo or whatever treatment they had, they knew they were going to get well. It was a requirement he had, that they believe the wellness was coming. And they did recover from cancer.

Love and miracles. Saints say that miracles are natural. One of my doctors has called me "a walking miracle."

Dr. Siegel refers to *A Course in Miracles*, and I think that's the basis of his therapy. To understand the Course better, it helps to attend a study group. While just reading the books, one's ego causes him to fall asleep, because it is threatened. The Course will question much of what you believe.

First I went to see Dr. Keith Vrehl and Jim Reese,

nutritionist, in the clinic in San Diego. Then I went to a doctor in North San Diego County who does aura reading or cleansing. He inspired me very much.

At my first acupuncture appointment, my sister and I went in and asked many questions. We wanted to find out what they thought was going to work. I believe you must take an active role and be interested in what's going on. I wanted to learn all I could about the alternative therapies.

I asked how acupuncture was going to help, and "what does this mean" and "what's that"? I took many notes. I really got educated quickly. After all this, I went back to Jim Reese and told him what I had decided to do. He seemed impressed by what I said. Most patients are not so motivated. He said that he could see that I would get well.

The only symptoms I had were the lesions. I've always been very energetic and strong. But all of a sudden there were these purple lesions on my arm. I had had plastic surgery on my nose, and when I went back for my six-month checkup, I showed the purple growths to the doctor who happened to be gay and a good friend.

He said he'd do a biopsy for me. He asked how I felt otherwise, and I told him, "fine." I had quit drinking about a year before almost completely and had changed my diet. I had been living a really wholesome, good life and had been reading literature on starting a business. I would sleep about six hours, then run around all day, going to auctions in the mornings. I was very active and very sharp.

After learning that I had Kaposi's sarcoma, I decided on alternative therapies, and took control of the treatments. My sister was there to help me monitor them. I made all the decisions, and she thought I made all the right ones. I did it myself. I was the one doing the controlling. Because it was my body, my thoughts...I was the one who had to do it. No one else could heal me. I was my own physician.

So it came down to a decision to live. There was a feeling,

a spirit in me, that said that I would be O.K., and after the therapies, I felt like a "million."

I thought, "This is ridiculous, how can I be sick? I'm far from it!" I realized I would get my healing.

I had growth on every level—mental, psychological, educational, spiritual. I was finding out who I really was. I was knowing the truth—sticking to the truth, telling the truth, and, of course, living the truth.

My life became very precious to me. I didn't have time to play or make a fool of myself. I had quite a few sessions of Rebirthing which helped me. I also had two Bach Flower Remedy treatments and a homeopathic treatment.

But the most important part of getting well was the spiritual growth. I was in remission eight months after I was diagnosed.

The lesions started shrinking after the first couple of weeks of fear and confusion—once I realized what alternative therapies were available and educated myself about them. I didn't have a doubt in my mind that I could heal myself.

And there's not a doubt in my mind that others can get well, too. It's a matter of educating themselves and acting on the information.

But many people with AIDS have a death wish. I know; I had felt suicidal at times when life wasn't going well—but not after my diagnosis.

Many people don't love themselves enough. Life is a schoolroom. If people do take their lives, they've got a lesson to learn and they will have to return and do life over until they do learn.

People don't believe in themselves. They give up so easily. They listen to the media. They become part of the statistics, because they actually believe that AIDS will kill them.

As Louise Hay says, you can live your life with ease, or you can live your life with dis-ease.

I've lost a couple of friends. Right from the start, they thought they were going to die. Their lifestyle, their belief system didn't change. They didn't know any better, I guess.

My old lifestyle included too much drinking on weekends; a poor diet; stress; recreational drugs about once a month—sniffing cocaine. I never smoked cigarettes, but until about ten years ago, I used to smoke pot off and on, maybe once or twice a week. I used to be sexually promiscuous. I feel that promiscuity may or may not be related to the disease. It may be transmitted through sexual activity, but I also believe that the disease is brought on by the thought that you're going to get it. Through guilt feelings, even small ones, you finally do get it, because thoughts are things, and powerful.

I feel that I brought the disease on. I did this by eating poor quality food, being sexually over-active, feeling I was unloved, and desiring attention.

My father hadn't known I was gay, but he found out soon after my AIDS diagnosis. I am very close to my mother now. In fact, she has just moved in with me. She's aware that I went through some heavy years of turmoil—actually, from about ages five to eleven. I had to take a look at why I had a speech impediment during these years, and why I was classified as being a slow learner. I am healing those old problems now.

It's amazing how bright children are, how they can put on a facade, and how they can create anything for attention!

During that time, I had two stepfathers who were alcoholic, and a much older stepbrother by whom I was molested sexually a great deal. Fortunately, my mother got a divorce. We moved to the country and I finally had her attention. I went from being a "C" student to an "A" student, and my speech impediment dropped away spontaneously, completely cleared up. I graduated from high school a year early and then went to college.

Also, from the time I was five years old I had a problem

with strep throat and infections. I was given heavy doses of antibiotics—penicillin, Septra, a couple of really heavy-duty ones. I had vaccines in the Army before overseas duty. A lot of antibiotics, and they made me sick.

I had a number of venereal diseases, some of them several times. It was life in the fast lane.

I had a great deal of energy, was highly motivated, so I was very active. Working in bars had something to do with it, too.

When I was drinking a lot, I'd tell myself, "You should stop drinking; you have no right to drink!" I could see that I wasn't handling the alcohol, and I started working on it. I had almost completely stopped drinking the year before my diagnosis, and since then, I don't drink at all.

I had been a vegetarian for two years when I was a teenager, and had felt really great then. I wanted to get back to it, and I did.

I had a general knowledge of a wholesome diet, but I had gone along with what everybody else did—got caught up in all of it—fast foods, liquor, etc.

In San Diego I had quite a reputation for being the funny guy. It was kind of stressful trying to keep everyone laughing.

In the early 80s, I felt very proud to be gay. I didn't flaunt it; I wasn't a typical gay. When AIDS started being publicized, I wasn't ashamed of being gay, but I didn't tell anyone I was. As far as I was concerned it was better left unsaid unless someone asked.

I was diagnosed about two days after I had opened up my flower business—a shop called "Exotic Flowers." Before that, in addition to being a bartender, I was a sales manager for about five years. I did much traveling as manager for a marketing company. I also was a retail manager for Saks Fifth Avenue, which was stressful, as I was supervising many employees.

So I worked very hard and I played very hard. As a sales

rep, my territory was from Palm Springs all the way up past San Francisco. Being on the road a lot, the only place I could socialize when I got off work was at a club, so I would do heavy drinking and heavy sex.

I still think, even if everyone says that AIDS is sexually transmitted, that I brought it on to get attention, too.

But now that I've recovered, I've learned to love myself, every moment. It's like the saying in Alcoholics Anonymous, "One day at a time." I live each day to the fullest, as if it were my last.

When my mother and I were having a deeply serious talk about dying from AIDS, she said, "You could die from this disease, or you could go out tomorrow and be hit by a car. So why don't you live each day to the fullest, not knowing when you'll go!" She said that's the attitude you should take.

I've learned to be calm. I do creative visualization, meditation, and spiritual mind treatments. It's knowing that everything is O.K. All is well, all is perfect in reality, and you can bring this perfection into manifestation.

I start my day and end it by surrendering and turning my life over to God. I'm not afraid to die, either, because I know that when I die, it's only the beginning of a new start, on a higher level. When I die, be it at 30 years or at 103 years, whatever the case may be, I will go when I'm supposed to.

Dr. Siegel points out in his book that some patients who are told they have six months to live, often die within a matter of weeks. No one has the right to play God. I don't think any doctor should tell a patient: "Well, you have about three or four months left." People believe their doctors. They believe that since the doctor has been educated, he knows. So they die. It's a self-fulfilling prophecy.

Dr. Siegel ran a test, where he used sugar water and told the patients this was the cure for their type of cancer. This placebo treatment worked in 75% of these cases. He found that all he had to do was simply to convince them. They believed him and lived. The tremendous power of the mind! Belief and faith determines life or death—it works both ways.

I had a brother-in-law who had leukemia. The doctors did a bone-marrow transplant from his twin sister and, even after they did all this surgery, he died at 33 years of age. My sister, who had been married to him since she was 16, told me, "You know, Doug, he was tired of fighting, and the night before he died, I knew he was going to go, from the way he said good-by."

He died of cardiac arrest. I had known Tim since I was about seven. He was a very bright man, and it hurt me that he finally just gave up. He chose when he was ready to go. We can do that. I believe that if I were ready to die, I'd just lie in my bed and in the morning I'd be dead. I could will myself to do that. Trained thought is much more powerful than untrained thought. And mankind has that power. The power of man's thought is amazing.

For the past year and a half, through Science of Mind, I've been training my thinking. I had a very good teacher, a master. She taught us how to put what we decide to do or have in Divine Mind, and that we can manifest it within 48 hours. We all have this power. It's a knowingness, and you accept the fact that you have the right, that it's your divine right, to have anything you want. As a whole, we're geared in this society to work very hard to get what we want. I don't work hard; I work smart.

It's knowing that you deserve—we all deserve—everything on this planet that we want. Our Creator didn't put it there for us to lack it, scratch for it, and suffer. We're here on earth to enjoy life, to have fun. I really think that God has great humor, and we're all taking life too seriously. I play as much as I can.

Children, from the time they're born, are told by parents, "no, don't, can't, shouldn't" to the point where they are stifled in their desires and capacities. When you look at little two-year-olds, you see in their eyes that they're not dumb. They are pure energy and power—until they are trained not to be. A little child is in communion with the Christ Child. A little child is going for everything because he knows he can—until he or she is told differently by an adult—someone who gives him/her that look and word of disapproval and limitation.

Science of Mind teaches that our minds are very powerful—tools we have been given to use. We can create health thoughts or sickness thoughts; both manifest outwardly.

For example: if you think "safe sex" is going to work it may, if it is safe, if you don't pass bodily fluids. But if you believe you can get AIDS by being in casual contact with somebody with AIDS, you're going to get it anyway. So "safe sex" depends on individuals and their thoughts. Personally, I don't do even "safe sex."

Another thing I've stopped doing is reading about all the different symptoms of AIDS patients, because I might accept them in my own mind, and thus create them in my body.

I know of one gentleman working with AIDS patients who created AIDS in himself—not through sexual transmission, but through manifesting it, starting with thought. I believe he wanted to impress people to get some attention. He was a psychotherapist, someone I thought would know better. This story shows that we're all very vulnerable when we don't control our thinking. We need to learn to control, to use, and to train our thoughts. Thoughts are very powerful. The negative thoughts we express carelessly can manifest negatively in our lives.

One word we use so much is "shouldn't." "I shouldn't have done that." "You shouldn't do that..." And "don't" and "can't"—they're all negative. And "That really kills me!" That phrase is a biggy; it can really kill you, if you keep saying it. Or, "I could just die for a piece of cake." That's a ridiculous statement.

We put these messages into our subconscious. If we

record them and they pass as universal law, they will follow through as manifestation. The universal law does not distinguish between what is good or bad for us. It picks up what we think and what is said, then it follows through. Universal law will bring it to you—good or bad —what you think, visualize and express in speech.

But you can train your thoughts and keep them on track. It's easy. Dr. Ernest Holmes' books are amazing; they teach you how to start training your thoughts. But some people don't want to educate themselves, train their thinking. Their ignorance is sad, because they could learn how to change their lives, become masters of them. Some of us get very comfortable in our mental patterns; they become hard to break. But they can kill us if we let them.

I had much to learn. I learned about the power of thought and was able to prove it to myself. I had to put it to the test immediately, because if I hadn't I would have died.

I'm not dead and I'm not going to die of AIDS. I'm in good health now.

I'm much more realistic about things. I tell myself the truth, I accept only the truth and what my truth is. There's no second-guessing. If I say something, I do it. I call it "completing." Time is too precious to waste with fooling myself or anybody else. I go right to the point.

My experience with AIDS has taught me that people can learn to heal themselves—through nutrition and through thought.

It's not only my disease that has been healed, but my relationships with people, including my parents. I've made quite a few new friends and enjoy my work immensely, too. Working with flowers is healing in itself.

I believe that what I've done can work for anyone. Once people get it into their minds to be truthful with themselves and learn what truth is, they can educate themselves as I have done. It can't help but work for them, too—it is a universal law.

Some people have the misconception that AIDS is a form of punishment from God. That's impossible. God doesn't punish anybody. We're all made in the image of God; why would he punish what he's made in his image? God doesn't want us to suffer; he wants only good for us. He is All Good.

We brought AIDS on ourselves, and we must get back to base—to home base with God. In the process of doing that, we heal ourselves.

I've always been a very positive person. I learned to laugh when most people might cry. That's not unrealistic. I extract the truth from the problem and ask myself: "How can I change this? Can it be changed? Am I willing to change it?"

I laugh a lot, love a lot. I'm a compassionate person. I love people and I love life. I stick to it. And I plan on being here for quite a long time. I want to help educate people. The *Course in Miracles* states it very well by saying that we're all teachers and we're all students. I want to share with others, including my young nieces and nephews, the experience of learning and teaching.

Your greatest fear is the thing you will create. Job in the Bible said, "The thing I greatly feared has come upon me." Fear is nothing, but we must learn that fear is nothing, that it has no power.

There's a saying, "When fear knocked on the door, I answered with faith and no one was there."

With faith, you can know that all will be well—your body, your life.

Just turn it all over to God.

And love yourself!

*   *   *   *   *

One year later:

During my illness, I saw a doctor in Los Angeles named Dr. Scolaro, who was most knowledgeable and gave me a great deal of help and support. My last blood test showed that the AIDS virus was isolated and is not now spreading through my body. The K.S. is also 80 percent gone.

I give credit to Dr. Scolaro and to my own self-healing practices and beliefs. I believe that AIDS is a call for humankind to learn how to love—for people to learn to love each other unconditionally and for each of us to love ourselves. I believe that you can't change the world for the better unless you stop and change yourself for the better. I've learned a valuable lesson about loving myself because of this AIDS virus. AIDS was given to me as a gift, a tool to learn more about myself, and really, to learn the greatest lesson in my life—how to LOVE.

WHAT DOUGLAS JOHNSON DID

• He decided that he did not have to die, but was prepared for death if it came.

• He took an active role in his healing, and discovered new healing methods.

• He refused the AZT drug treatment that was offered him.

• He discovered holistic and spiritual healing. The combination of natural therapies and spiritual inspirations worked for him.

• He was encouraged and inspired by the books

he read, especially *A Course in Miracles* and *Science of Mind* books.

• He had a supportive family, especially his sister.

• With her help, he studied alternatives to the drug treatments that allopathic medicine was offering him.

• They took control of the decisions as to how the natural treatments would be used.

• He was a very positive person. When friends would cry about his disease, he could laugh.

• He changed his destructive lifestyle.

• He improved his diet, reduced stress, stopped sexual promiscuity, and the over-consumption of alcohol.

• Before the diagnosis, he had worked and played too hard. After it, he learned to slow down.

• He developed an inward calm and knew that everything would come out harmoniously.

• He does not accept doctors' diagnoses such as "Only one year to live."

• He believed in the power of the will—that a

person can will himself to health or almost anything else.

• He studies, believes in, and practices the teachings of "The Science of Mind."

• He learned that everyone deserves all the good he or she wants and that it is obtainable.

• He declares, "We were not put here on earth to suffer."

• He believes that a sense of humor is important, and says "Most people are too serious." He plays whenever he can.

• He doesn't believe in "safe sex" as it is defined today.

• He learned that "thoughts are things," that thoughts are very powerful.

• He learned that negative thoughts expressed carelessly will manifest in some kind of negative experience. Words and thoughts are important and powerful.

• He learned that mankind must learn to retrain its thinking, and that trained thinking is much more powerful than untrained thinking.

• He tells himself the truth, and only the truth.

- His relationships with people in his life have been healed.

- His experience with AIDS has taught him this: people can heal themselves through nutrition and with thought.

- He always asks himself: "How can I change it?"

- He laughs much.

- He is compassionate toward others.

- He loves people.

- Douglas Johnson loves life.

Love, Medicine, & Miracles

Dr. Siegel reveals a remarkable insight into the human mind and its astonishing capacity for healing the body. What is unusual is that a medical doctor would do research in this field of self-healing.

Love, Medicine & Miracles is an inspiring best seller, acclaimed by members of the scientific community for its candid honesty and use of real case studies.

The authors highly recommend it, but point out that self-healing of the body can take place WITHOUT the chemotherapy and other harsh medical treatments. At this point in our history, patients in hospitals are not allowed to use the mind only. Perhaps someday that will come!

Revelations on healing in this "New Age" will lead both doctors and patients to this higher point. We still have far to go, but work like Dr. Siegel's are indications that the dawn of a New Age is here.

Dr. Siegel is not only saying, "Patient, help heal thyself!", but also advising the patients to say, "Look, God, I can't take care of this one, you'll have to handle it."

For a medical doctor to think and act in this manner is truly revolutionary. "New Age" concepts — natural therapies, inspiration, the power of the mind, God as Healer — are beginning to penetrate the medical monolith. —B.L.

Note: The book *Love, Medicine & Miracles*, two audio tapes and a two-hour video cassette with Dr. Siegel are available.

Jeffrey Joshua Migota, R.N.

Jeffrey Migota is a most unusual man—an outstanding representative of a New Age person. A Registered Nurse, he personifies the best in that demanding and unselfed career. He is compassionate and goes far beyond the call of duty.

Because of his spiritual orientation, Jeffrey Migota exudes an aura of divine helpfulness. Here is an example, in his own words.

"A woman came into the ward last night, unable to walk, with a painful ankle. As soon as I could find time, I treated her with aura massage. This is a therapeutic 'touch' without actually touching the body. Meditating while doing so, I passed my hand over the painful part of the body, in the 'aura field.' After twenty minutes, the pain vanished. It did not return, and she could walk."

It is remarkable that Jeffrey can do this type of healing in the setting where he works—the Emergency Room of the

Washington Hospital Center, a large hospital in D.C. This is the most demanding of all nursing environments.

Jeffrey is a man of slight stature and weight, but he finds an energy in himself beyond the physical, to help the unfortunate people who come into Emergency. The desire to help and heal motivates his life.

Jeffrey's mother died in childbirth when he was born. There were older brothers and sisters. Many years later, after he became an R.N., he learned that his mother had wanted one of her children to become a nurse. None of his siblings selected this profession, but Jeffrey, the youngest, did—without knowing his mother's wish.

Jeffrey enrolled in a nursing class at Prince George's Community College and Maryland University. It started out with ten men and 100 women; eight men and 60 women graduated. Few males choose nursing as a career. However, the percentage of males entering the nursing profession is increasing. Jeffrey Migota graduated in 1979.

Jeffrey Migota's Adventure

I am a Registered Nurse; I am also a survivor of AIDS. Even though I have been trained in the medical field, I am positive that Holistic Medicine is the strongest aid in fighting AIDS!

(The root meaning of the word "medicine" does not refer to drugs. It means "the healing art.")

During my own journey of conquering AIDS, I have been asked by quite a few persons, "How can you be a Registered Nurse, giving pills, injections, and using Western medicine, when you yourself practice Holistic Healing?"

Nursing is much more than giving someone a pill or taking a blood pressure. To me, nursing is nurturing, listening, and caring for those with whom I come in contact, including family and friends. A touching hand, with an open ear, quite often does more than a so-called "magic" pill or shot.

When I entered the nursing profession in 1977 as a technician, I alternated between Emergency Room Nursing and Hospice (Home for Dying) Nursing. I learned at Hospice, through nursing many cancer and terminal patients that their will to live and inner strength plus positive thinking outweighed the effects of chemotherapy and radiation. I have seen some miraculous recoveries from cancer in people the doctors thought were "death row" patients.

I wouldn't trade nursing for any other profession or any amount of money. It has given me so much understanding of people.

I only regret that I cannot give more individual attention to my patients. With only five or six nurses on duty and 75 or more patients on our shift alone, it is very difficult. Please remember, I'm dealing in a very stressful environment, where gunshot wounds, overdoses, heart attacks, and strokes are an ongoing process 24 hours a day.

I see ten or more AIDS people during a weekend period. Some are very depressed, some in the final stages of life (by their choice, I regretfully add). To hold their hands, listen to their fears, "to just be," is an opportunity and gift that only God could bestow upon me.

There is a lot of stress for me and at times I have too much sympathy, but that is what they need. If I can give them a little hope and cheer, then it is all worth it.

I believe that stress is a co-factor that lowers the immune system, so I must always keep myself one step ahead of it. This is where a simple meditation and a protective shield of white light go a long way for me.

For those who do not understand what I mean by a protective white light: the energy field around your body is known as your aura. This aura can protect you from physical harm, sickness, or danger. By creating more energy around you, you can create an energy field that helps to ward off anything that may be physically harmful to you. To make it sound simpler, it's like putting a non-penetrable dome around you for protection and strength.

These extremely stressful conditions at the hospital were a problem for me but I learned to deal with them. Ellie Kierson, my meditation guide, knew I was having problems at the hospital where I work only on weekends. I do what they call the Weekend Alternative (one works 12 hours on Saturday and 12 hours on Sunday and gets paid for 40 hours). I would come home Monday mornings from work a total wreck because of the way some of the nurses treat the AIDS people and all the negative remarks that I would hear. Ellie taught me how to do meditations and protect myself with a "white light". She created a meditation tape for me. In a stressful situation I break away quickly and put on this tape. After listening for a few minutes, I return to the floor as if nothing had happened. It works really well for me.

I found these New Age holistic healing techniques after I contracted AIDS. They helped me conquer it, and I am grateful that I can help myself and others with this new knowledge.

I always try to remember that in order to be loved, to be helped and to be cared for, I must first GIVE... for by giving love, help and care, I can truly receive them back, tenfold.

How I Conquered AIDS

I fell sick with AIDS, but I conquered it—with a combination of natural therapies, changing my lifestyle in every possible way to a healthful one, transforming my thinking, my consciousness, and following a spiritual path.

Getting AIDS and conquering it has meant great mental and spiritual growth for me. One of the first and most important facts I learned was, and I quote from Mary Baker Eddy: ..."mortal mind is the cause of all disease. Destroy the mental sense of the disease, and the disease itself disappears. Destroy the sense of sin, and sin itself disappears."[1]

I was fortunate to meet a man in Saudi Arabia who was also an R.N. He was a student of Christian Science, became a good friend, and introduced me to this spiritual science. I am learning divine truths about life through the Christian Science textbook, which I read daily. It is *Science and Health with Key to the Scriptures,* by Mary Baker Eddy. This inspired author reintroduced to humanity the spiritual healing that Christ Jesus and others of Biblical days performed. They knew that God, Divine Love, is able to heal our sicknesses, and without drugs or other material methods. These eternal truths are available to us today, resulting in more healthful and happy lives, more peace and love in individual lives and hence in the world.

Through my experience with AIDS, I learned to receive as well as give. I have always been a giver. When a person calls to say he needs help, I'm always there. But I would never let anyone know when I was hurting; I've had difficulty in asking or receiving.

However, I feel that in the last few years, and especially the last few months, I have learned to turn to other people and say, "I hurt." This March (1988) was the second anniversary of the death of my lover, and I let people know I was hurting. I needed the comfort that others could give, and it really did help me. So that is another lesson I have learned.

Before going into details, I want to state that I have been free from AIDS now for three years. The first time I was hospitalized was in February/March of 1983. For one year I took AL 721 and Naltrexone. My last hospital stay was in July, 1985. From that date on, I took no medications of any kind for AIDS, adopted natural and spiritual therapies, and have felt well, with abundant energy to do my work, from that time until this.

I had gone overseas to Saudi Arabia to work as a Registered Nurse in February, 1983 for an American company contracted to the Saudi government. It was during this time, in a period of four months (March through June, 1983), that I developed six bouts of pneumonia, getting progressively worse each time. Finally, during the fifth or sixth episode, a sputum culture was obtained and a diagnosis of *Pneumocystis carinii* pneumonia (PCP) was made; this was in May or June of 1983.

What do I think causes AIDS? I believe there are various causes for the HIV virus or the dis-ease, ranging from exposure to Hepatitis B and the serum used in the Hepatitis B testing in the late 1970s; the overuse of antibiotics over the years; all the pills that are forced into us at different times; destructive lifestyles (drug use, a variety of sexual partners, poor nutrition, etc.); previous syphilis and/or gonorrhea; the polluted environment—the air, the water and the chemicalized food; a poor mental attitude and low self-esteem. All these factors add to a depressed immune system. When one becomes exposed to the virus while the resistance is low, he can get the disease.

In my own case, however, I have never had any of these addictions nor any venereal disease; surely that freedom helped me conquer this dis-ease.

There is much publicity on the transmission of AIDS as primarily sexual. I have wondered how I contracted it, as I never was sexually promiscuous. Larry, my partner/lover for 24 years, died in March, 1986 of this dis-ease. Whether he transmitted it to me or I to him is not the point. We do not know how long this virus can lie dormant in a human body.

May I explain my use of the word "dis-ease." "Dis" means reversal or lack of, and "ease" means comfort or freedom from discomfort, so "dis-ease" is basically a state of being without comfort. And that is what illness is. But "ease" or "dis-ease" are not only material states. There are important mental/ psychological/spiritual factors also, that play significant roles in one's state of well-being, or lack thereof.

I also feel that a lack of any spiritual nature helps the disease progress. I had drifted away from the Catholic Church in which I was raised, and had lost contact with my inner or spiritual self. But now I feel that I am in contact with God constantly, as God is within, and it is not necessary to be a part of an organized religion to be God-conscious. To believe in God or be in contact with this Divine Power, one does not need an intermediary. One can reach God or Universal Spirit, directly. There is a vast difference between spirituality and religion. A highly developed spiritual sense gives one complete control and a tremendous power over all manifestation.

One must consider his entire being—mental, spiritual, and physical. One needs to learn about nutrition. Doctors and the schools teach little on this important subject. Television misinforms us; its principal aim is to sell products for its advertisers, with no concern whether these products are good or bad for the public. So each person is on his own; he must cultivate learning and educate himself, for survival.

I learned about the chemical Biphenyl. This is a substance that is used in the embalming process in mortuaries, but is also used to embalm citrus fruits, to "keep them fresh," as they say. The F.D.A. states that these chemicals won't harm you as the quantities are so small. But when you consider that we eat them day after day—all these "small quantities" put into our beautiful bodies over the years adds up to pounds of these poisons affecting us. Foods in cans and cartons often list chemicals as part of the ingredients, "to preserve freshness." These chemicals prolong shelf life, but some are carcinogenic agents. [2]

Once I wondered why the cancer and other degenerative disease rates were increasing so much; now I believe I have found the answer.

I have purified my diet and my lifestyle. To the best of my ability at present, I have tried to increase my physical, mental, and spiritual well-being.

I believe that by neglecting or abusing the body, a person is asking for some type of illness or dis-ease. But if he considers his body to be a temple of God, as I do, he will want to improve the quality and appearance of the temple on a daily basis.

I was created by the Lord in his image, as it says in Genesis, the first book of the Bible. My body was originally pure and clean. And that is true of everyone. In the beginning, what did God give Adam and Eve in the Garden to eat? Fruits, vegetables and nuts. He did not give them animals to eat, and the air and water didn't contain any contaminants or pollutants. The original state of man was health and happiness. Mankind has truly hurt itself with its fast, modern living and abuse of the body in every imaginable way. I try to treat my body well and take care of myself. Everyone should do the same.

Try to remember the main reason for eating—to nourish the body. It is not for mere pleasure. So, if something is made by factories to taste good, don't eat it for that reason. Ask yourself: "Is this food good for me, good for the health of my body?" Actually, the simple gifts of Nature taste the best, to the uncorrupted taste buds.

You don't need to eat the innocent and harmless creatures of God. They have their own reason for existence; that reason is not to satisfy a corrupted palate. Consider this: the animals' dead bodies do not reproduce, but when you pick the fruit from a tree or a vegetable from the plant, it reproduces itself from seeds. Doesn't this tell you something?

Consider all the steroids and antibiotics that are fed to livestock (to fatten them faster), and all the preservatives that are used in packaged foods. These do nothing but harm our health. This is why I stress the importance of a diet such as mine—fresh salads and other vegetarian foods, organic if possible. These foods cleanse the body instead of polluting it.

You will find yourself so healthy by eating fruits, vegetables, sprouts, and nuts that, in time, you'll wonder what you ever saw in meats, other animal products, and packaged foods prepared in factories.

Back in the 60s, I was about 230 pounds, but then I had stomach surgery, and lost 100 pounds. I have maintained that weight (135 pounds) since then. The surgery was a sub-total gastrectomy, where three-fourths of my stomach was removed. The following year doctors did a vagotomy—a procedure where the vagus nerve is clipped because it is secreting too much hydrochloric acid. This was serious surgery, but I recuperated beautifully, and this surgery led me to better nutrition.

I have never liked, and have hardly ever eaten, fried foods—French fries, fried chicken, etc. Just the thought of all that cooked grease is repellent to me. A fried hamburger with French fries is one of the worst things one can eat. I am grateful that my doctors taught me years ago how bad cooked grease would be for my stomach condition. So I have maintained this grease-free diet for the past 25 years or so.

I am almost a vegetarian now. I never ate much meat, and now there is no meat in my diet. I eat fruit, vegetables, sprouts, and nuts, but no boxed, canned, or packaged foods. Made in factories, these are dead foods; they have very little life-sustaining nutrition in them.

I eat some fish, but now I am concerned about fish because of the contaminated waters. I drink no tap water, only spring water, and no sodas of any kind.

I don't stuff myself while eating. For health, it is important not to overeat.

By eating natural foods (foods grown by natural processes without any chemicals being added) I live as close to nature as possible. I thought of going on a macrobiotic diet, but have not done so because of the weight loss in the beginning of the program. So what I have done is to take a little information from macrobiotics, some from the vegetarian philosophy, and created my own diet. It seems to be working quite well for me.

The whole time I was overseas, I maintained my daily vitamin therapy and kept up my nutritious diet. Over there, one eats a lot of beans, vegetables, fruits—and all naturally grown by local residents. I also did much jogging and swimming, as there was nothing else to do. These are some of the factors that saved me, I am sure. I was in the northern part of Saudi Arabia, in a desert town call Tabuk near the Lebanon border. The summertime temperature was 140 degrees, daily. Someone who has not lived there cannot imagine what it is like.

Co-Factors in AIDS

Promiscuity is certainly a co-factor in this disease. But remember, there are the IV drug users (who may or may not also be promiscuous), and also an increase in numbers of women, children, and other persons receiving blood transfusions who were never promiscuous. It may be, as stated in the book *Conquering AIDS Now!* that the bloodstream of humanity has become polluted. At first, all this pollution was outside of ourselves, and now it is within.

I am starting to believe that AIDS as well as many other dis-eases and illnesses are actually acquired by the body in response to something the body is trying to tell or teach us. I am not saying that I asked to be sick, but I let my body and mind accept illness.

I was sickly as a child and had a disease of the stomach or ulcers since I was twelve years old. Finally, when I was sixteen, the doctors did the surgery that I described earlier. I had always been susceptible to colds and minor viruses.

In my late teens, I discovered and used vitamins, good nutrition, and meditation. I think these helped build up my depleted immune system. But, as we all tend to do at times, I let myself go lax—three to four years prior to contracting this dis-ease.

I never had hepatitis B, the more serious form, but did have hepatitis A. I was treated with antibiotics over the years, but never penicillin, as I am allergic to it. Today, I feel that seven to ten days' treatment with antibiotics is too much, and I refuse to take any form of these drugs. But when I had my stomach surgery back in the 60s and also when I was in Saudi Arabia, with my many episodes of pneumonia, antibiotics were used.

Also, since I am a nurse and am exposed to many people in the Emergency Room who have hepatitis A and B, I have been given the Immune Globulin vaccination, which is, of course, derived from human plasma, a blood product. My hepatitis A, which I had back in 1965, was self-regulating. The doctor placed me on a high protein diet and bed rest. I took no medications, only vitamins.

I do not use recreational drugs. I tried smoking pot once many years ago but it made me sick, so I never tried it again. The same happened with poppers—I got headaches and became sick to my stomach. I took amphetamines a couple of times, especially when I was in college, but I didn't like the high, out-of-control feeling, and hated the coming down off it. So, beyond this, I have not experimented with drugs, and have no intentions of doing so. I can easily get high through my friendships, my meditations, and the resultant inner happiness.

About Celibacy

My lifestyle has changed dramatically since I recovered from AIDS. I have become celibate, basically for more than two years. Why? I don't want to take a chance of spreading the virus to someone else, which to me is the same as premeditated murder. Of course, there is "safe sex", so-called (rubbers and such things), but I don't believe those give 100% protection, and I would really feel and BE guilty, if I passed AIDS on to someone. So I stay away from sex now, even though I am convinced I have recovered from AIDS. Perhaps I am going through a phobic phase in sex, but I don't want to take any chances, in case there are some, for spreading this illness.

I do miss having a sexual relationship/partner, I can't deny that. Maybe someday I will be able to deal with it, but not at the present time. I have too many more important matters to attend to on behalf of my physical well-being and my spiritual growth.

But what does a person do about his sexual drives in cases like this? I remember asking a priest, years ago, what he did about his sexual drives, since celibacy is the order of the church for priests. "I pray about it. I ask God to help me," he replied. Others besides priests can do the same. Sexual appetites can be controlled by the mind and the will. Each one must choose between self-restraint and self-indulgence.

Do I feel I am still vulnerable? I feel that as long as I am alive, I am vulnerable. That's true of anyone. But as long as I keep up my positive attitude, stay away from prescribed drugs/medications, keep my diet as natural and vegetarian as possible, I believe that I will continue to be well.

Aspects of Holistic Healing

I am constantly seeking and experimenting with alternative treatments and therapies. At present I am with a "positive immunity" support group here in Washington, D.C. It is full of love, support for each other, and a constant flow of new ideas. From being strangers to each other, we have grown to love each other as brothers, mentally and spiritually. Our group is headed by a beautiful woman named Ellie Kierson. During the past three months or so, we have been exposed to different aspects of Holistic Healing: chiropractic, acupuncture, herbology, meditation. Ellie herself does guided imagery and Reiki. She is helping the group considerably and we're all very happy to have her with us. I joke with her, saying: "I hope your husband doesn't get too jealous about his wife spending three or four hours per week with 'her boys.'" She is very supportive and tends to meet each of our individual needs.

Conquering AIDS—
a Source of Life Transformation

My thinking about myself has been one of my greatest changes, and it has not been an easy road. The tired old expression "I'm dying with AIDS" was changed long ago for me to "I'm living with AIDS," and now I feel I can say "I've recovered from or conquered AIDS." The illness has taught me so much about life, love, and caring for myself as well as others. At times I feel truly spiritually lifted/gifted. I can't begin to describe the tremendous life experiences I am now having. In a way I am grateful for having had this disease, as it has opened up complete awareness to me. I have become involved in more constructive things than I would have done if I had remained healthy. Louise Hay, in her healing/teaching/training, is showing us how to love ourselves, our bodies, our inner souls.

I always was critical of myself, not pleased with my looks or my hair or something or other. I always indulged in much self-criticism. But now I am learning that I am the way I am, and it is O.K. I can look into the mirror now and tell myself that I do love that person who is looking back. I still have a long way to go, but I never stop working on it. By doing this, I can look at other people and share my love with them. I have been truly reaching out to others, trying to help them the best ways I can.

"Sweet are the uses of adversity," wrote the great Shakespeare. Troubles can be stepping stones to progress. It's all up to us. AIDS has really changed my life for the positive.

Being sick—and my recovery—have helped increase my awareness. I've become more aware of my health, of nutrition, of loving and of the potentials of spirituality.

I have never been as close to my family as now. My parents are deceased, but I have three sisters and one brother, all older than I. They were and are very supportive—not only with my identity crisis of some 25 years ago, but now with this dis-ease.

I consider other people's feelings much more now than I did before. I won't argue with anyone. If someone has something to say, whether I agree or disagree, I accept it, for that is his opinion and his right and I don't have time for disagreement or bad feelings in my life. I want to be at peace with myself, with others and, of course, the Lord, as He exists for me.

I'm more aware of my surroundings. More aware of little things that wouldn't have affected me in the past. Recently one of our nurses had her house burn down. I was on the phone immediately, saying, "You're welcome to stay here. Do you need money or clothes for the children?" I tend now to reach out very rapidly. This really has brought a new awareness to me of caring for others more.

My bout with AIDS has not hindered me professionally, but remember, I am a Registered Nurse working in an Emergency Room. About a year ago, one of the nurses left to work in another department after being in the E. R. and also knowing me for ten years. She had such a phobia about AIDS, afraid that she was going to get it, that (I believe) she left the E. R. in great fear of getting the disease from me by simply being in my environment.

Everyone at work knows that I am gay (although non-practicing at this time). Believe it or not, they figure that all gays either have AIDS or will come down with the dis-ease. This is a phobia and not a fact. The medical people are really uneducated on the subject of AIDS.

I have found that I have high energy for my demanding job, and in the past year I lost only seven days from work.

This is the first time in over 18 months that I haven't had the flu or a cold. Usually every winter I would come down with a cold or the flu at least four or five times, but I've gone through this entire winter well, and we've had a rather bad winter here.

It is interesting, how people who hear about my AIDS relate to me. Some cry, others hug me; most have sympathy and want to do anything and everything they can, but feel helpless. Well, I make it quite clear that I am not dying and having had this diagnosis doesn't put me or anyone else on The Last Road. I tell them that my life now is no different from theirs, and I am not crying over whether they might have a car accident or whatever in the next few days, so why cry over me? Once I explain this, people relate to me very well. In fact, most people have gotten much closer to me on different levels.

My Health History

When I was in Saudi Arabia and was so ill, they wanted to send me back to the States within the first six months, but I was too weak and too sick to travel. I couldn't even ambulate on my own. They had to tube me for awhile, which is no fun. That's when the term PCP first hit me. But while still in the States I had constant bouts of colds and pneumonia. Doctors kept telling me that I had a weak middle lobe and weak lower right lobe in my lungs, and kept giving antibiotics. I was also given antibiotics overseas.

But now I am against antibiotics, as I feel that we have been given too many of them. Besides, our bodies over a period of time build up a resistance to some antibiotics; certain bacterial/viral infections are no longer destroyed by the antibiotics we once used; the viruses have built up a tolerance.

I have had repeated tests done over the past two years. It's been over two years since my last HIV antibody testing, but

I have my T-Cell counts done about once a month. The lowest my count has ever gone down to was 290. In August 1988, it rose to 670, which is on the healthy side of normal. I credit my rise in my T-Cell count strictly on alternative methods, my attitude and not on anything my doctor did.

However, I do not feel that T-Cell monitoring is a good parameter. The count can change from day to day. I have people with counts in the 300s-400s who are very ill in the hospital, while a friend who tested 7 on his last count is as healthy as I am.*

In Saudi Arabia

Saudi Arabia seems to have no problem with AIDS in its own population. To the best of my knowledge, I was the only Person With AIDS at that time. Since returning to the States, I have heard of three other Americans I worked with over there dying from AIDS and at least another four or five with positive HIV status. I wish I had known sooner and had gotten to them; perhaps I could have helped. Well, it's too late for them probably. May they rest in peace and enjoy being true spirits now.

My AIDS Condition in Saudi Arabia

My illness first manifested while I was in Saudi Arabia. The early symptoms included severe fatigue, extreme night sweats, fevers as high as 105°, anorexia, weight loss (about ten pounds), diarrhea. You name the symptom and I had it. I spent almost the first five months in Saudi Arabia in the hospital being treated for these symptoms. On one occasion I ran a 105° fever for four or five days and my family here in the U.S. was

---

* One explanation of this is that no one knows what the T-Cell count was before the illness.

notified of my impending death. I was lucky to escape brain damage.

To get my fevers down in the hospital, they gave me aspirin. They didn't use ice packs or thermic blankets. I told them I wanted Tylenol and fluids. "Give me IV fluids, fluids to drink, anything," and that's what they did. I kept my room very cool even though I was freezing, but I wanted my body temperature to drop, so the air conditioner was kept on cool.

Oxygen was given to me for comfort a few times via nasal cannula at between two to three liters, but it was not part of my regime, as oxygen tends to give me headaches. Not having oxygen on a regular basis probably was a good thing. I guess I am thankful that Saudi Arabia is somewhat behind in Western medical techniques and that my early symptoms happened in the Middle East. If they had happened here in the States and Western medical practices such as drugs and oxygen had been given to me, I might not be alive today to share my experience with you.

Dr. Saiid Baidas, a doctor in Saudi Arabia, first diagnosed me. After so many bouts of pneumonia and exhibiting the other symptoms, he finally did a sputum culture. He also did a spinal tap as he thought I might have spinal meningitis because of the high fever and highly elevated white count. The sputum culture came back; the result was PCP. I didn't know what this type of pneumonia was or that it was a diagnosis for AIDS until I came back to the States in 1985. I was given antibiotics which came from Sweden, Denmark, and England; I was not told their names.

I was very naive about this dis-ease. You must keep in mind that newspapers, current events, and anything else that might be happening in the world don't necessarily get to the Middle East. They print only what they wish to.

Another doctor from Canada, (James Wensney, M.D.), said that since I was gay and had come from the States, he suspected that I had what was becoming known as AIDS. He took a sample of my blood and sent it off to England where testing was being done. I assume it was the ELISA only, since I don't think the Western Blot was being done yet. (Now the ELISA is given first. If antibodies are present, the Western Blot is given as a follow-up to confirm the ELISA.) I tested HIV positive. I feel that I probably had the HIV virus for at least one or two years prior to the full-blown symptoms that developed in early 1983.

I was very sick. After the first bout of pneumonia, I began to get better for about a week to ten days. Then I started going downhill. I always knew when I was getting sick as I'd start losing my appetite, and for me this is a bad sign. Then I would get diarrhea, fever, and usually after two or three days of this, I would have to go to the hospital due to dehydration and increased anorexia. I would get dry heaves due to my stomach being empty of any solids. In Egypt I went through a bad stage which started gradually. I'd be out to dinner and would have trouble eating and when I would look at the food I'd get sick. Eventually the sight of a glass of water would cause me to have dry heaves and I knew I was in big trouble. About five days after this started, I was in a bad state of malnutrition and dehydration. The diagnosis was anorexia nervosa.

I spent a month with a psychiatrist there. This happened when Larry, my lover, told me on the phone that he was dying of AIDS. The news that my father had died that same week was too much for me to deal with. But I told the psychiatrist I was going to recover from this and I did.

I started gradually with water, just sips. They had been giving me hyperalimentation (food lipids through IV) and I finally told them to stop this treatment as I felt this was something I had to do on my own, to face my own depression over the bad news and restore my own mental and physical health.

I feel that the climate I lived in was helpful. The air is not polluted as it is here. There are natural vegetables and fruits and the lifestyle is strict there. I don't give credit for my healing to the antibiotics that I received because I feel that the PCP can be cleared up without them. Because of the high fevers and the dehydration, I did take what was given me and drank a lot of fluids. I insisted that I get daily vitamins and the doctor met my demands. Vitamin C and beta-carotene were also important. So there were the vitamins, the fluids, the clean air, my positive attitude, and the spiritual treatment. I feel I survived because of all these factors.

I refused to take the psychotropic drugs as I didn't want anyone playing with my mind except myself. The doctor was really furious with me, but I held my ground. I was so bad that I was hearing voices and constant music and I thought that perhaps I was going crazy, but I was determined to overcome this and I did.

I never heard anyone talking about my condition or that I might die. There was an inner voice, my inner self (spirit/soul) telling me that I did not have to die from this dis-ease, that yes, I was very sick, but I would recover. Then, after returning to the States, it was emphasized to me in the New Age movement that AIDS does not have to be a death sentence and the more I heard that, the more I was sure that what I had felt or heard before was my spirit directing me.

From the onset, I told myself that "I'm not going to die from this dis-ease because it doesn't have to be that way." During the nine years I've been a nurse and the previous two years I spent working in a hospice, I have taken care of and listened to many cancer patients. This was a good learning process for me. I saw many of these "terminal" patients recover through their own therapies, positive thinking, diet changes, etc.

I never believed that I would die from the illness, but a couple of times I was ready to give up and give in to the illness because of the loss of my loved one. A year ago, I even attempted suicide, but I reached out quickly and got help. It had nothing to do with the dis-ease. The dis-ease has never frightened me, but I missed and still miss the person I was with for so many years that when he was gone after one year, I just couldn't accept it. I've come a long way since then and I've accepted Larry's death and realize that this is a part of life that I have to face.

The healing process has been nothing but progress for me. But if I had listened to my doctor in the States, I'm almost positive that I would either be in a hospital now on a respirator or perhaps even dead. My doctor still wants me on AZT, Acyclovir, the TB vaccine and who knows what else, but my answer is NO and will continue to be NO.

Feeling Like a Social Outcast

When I got AIDS, I did feel like this, but despite the ignorance, hysteria and prejudice of others around me, I knew in my heart that I had to try to prove myself. I felt different and like an outcast, but I think that almost every gay person experiences this particular feeling sometime in his life, especially when first discovering he is, shall we say, "different."

What really helped me to accept myself was this: in Cairo, I was living in a suburb called Maadi, which is not far from the leper colony. I would go there quite often to give support, love or whatever I could. I learned that lepers, too, are human and are beautiful people. They weren't going to spread their infection to me (regardless of what many medical theories say). I would walk around with them, and I kept thinking to myself, "Why do they have to be colonized and put into these living conditions?" It is a fear of contagion on the part of others. So I made a commitment to myself that I would not let myself be considered an outcast.

I show and extend love and a true concern for people. No one ever looks at me as being a sick person. I don't look it, but even if I did, I don't think anyone would even notice, as they would be looking at me from a different viewpoint—of friendship, love and caring—returning to me the qualities that I am sending out.

About Judging Gays With AIDS

Some of the religious people are talking about punishment that is "deserved." Do you tell a person dying from cancer that he/she is being punished for what he has done? I do feel that I needed this disease and permitted myself to contact it for many reasons and for many lessons that I needed to learn.

What is judgment? Each person must judge himself. I don't believe that anyone has a right to judge another. And you know how the Bible tells about Judgment Day, in which all will be revealed about oneself and there will be no hiding. I believe that I will be that Judge. The Spirit, that inner God within, knows all that I have done and when that glorious day comes, there is no way that I can hide from myself.

My Lover Larry—AIDS & DEATH

I returned to the States to take care of my lover, Larry. He had remained here and when he called me to say he was dying from AIDS, I immediately returned. I didn't know anything about this dis-ease, so I conferred with his doctors, who are well known in the States for their work in infectious diseases. I asked them to explain exactly what this disease is, the ways of catching it, etc. I even attended medical seminars to educate myself.

These doctors had Larry on Acyclovir, an anti-viral drug. After about six months of continued use, he started having grand mal seizures. I looked up Acyclovir in the PDR (Physicians Desk Reference) and learned that one of the long-term use side effects was seizures. I immediately stopped giving Larry the drug and the doctors started screaming at me that he needed the drug. At this time, which was his worst three months of living, I told the doctors I would rather have him sick and die naturally from this dis-ease than to continue having these grand mal seizures. By this time, Larry had become a total bed patient, with loss of all bodily functions, and his mind had started to slip away.

The doctors also had him on various types of antibiotics. He had PCP twice, and continuous thrush and various other ailments. He ended up dying of meningitis, PCP and quite a few other dis-eases. Did all those antibiotics, etc. help him? NO! I have friends on AZT and they ask me "should I continue or quit it?" I don't like to give my personal opinion. I merely tell them: "Whatever you choose to do or feels right for you," but I myself will never, never take it. I have watched individuals coming into the Emergency Room who are on AZT and need blood transfusions. I ask: "How long have you been on AZT?", and usually it's six months and then the transfusions are needed. I don't feel that any of these drugs are helping them; they only give added time, and a poor quality of time. These drugs seem to cause them to just waste away. So for me, no drugs.

I feel that those who don't survive this dis-ease are people who have given up hope. That's what my lover did. I put him on megavitamins, but it was too late.

I even had a Christian Science practitioner speak with him regarding spiritual healing, but Larry refused to stop taking the drugs, which is a requirement for Christian Science treatment. The practitioner tried to convince Larry to stop the drugs and said that he would work with him through the Christ power, but Larry said "NO." He felt that Western medicine and his doctors were right. But not one drug that Larry took ever made him better. The thrush continued, the night sweats and fevers increased and his dementia got worse. All he did was go downhill. It is my conviction that his cooperation with Western medicine was his biggest downfall and prevented recovery.

Some people are stronger physically or mentally, and some are weaker. Much depends on how open one is to new ideas and alternative treatments. In Larry's case, he was weak when it came to drug use. When I was overseas, he started to get involved with all kinds of drugs. He took uppers/downers, sniffed coke, used poppers (amylnitrate),* and drank a lot of alcohol. At the same time while getting high, he was also running around and becoming promiscuous.

As we are learning more and more each day, these drugs are immuno-suppressive.* Many people are ruining their lives with these drugs and cheap lifestyles.

I wish more people knew that they have other options. If you can instill the thought of other options into their minds while they're still capable of rational thought, that thought will start to expand and eventually hit their brain causing pictures to start flashing. They'll be more open and may try meditation, prayer, spiritual treatment, acupuncture, vitamin therapy, colonics, homeopathic medication or other holistic therapies that are available to us, by our own choice. Many of these persons hear of these treatments too late, or they're just too ingrained with the concepts of Western medicine. We must forget the thought of a "magic silver bullet" that will cure all ills. We must try to get through to those who are still suffering without knowing they have other options.

This book, *THEY CONQUERED AIDS!* is very important, and should reach millions of desperate people in the world who need to learn about Holistic Healing.

---

* AUTHORS' NOTE:
Amylnitrate ("poppers") may be the original cause or trigger of the AIDS syndrome in the gay population. Widespread use of "poppers" by homosexuals began shortly before AIDS appeared in the late 1970's. It has been suggested to the authors that amylnitrate reduces the activity of the center of the brain which regulates the white blood cells. This "high" in the brain tells the body that "all is well;" therefore, the body does not produce more white blood cells. Other drugs also cause immuno-suppression of the body's defenses, but amylnitrate is especially harmful because the vapors of the drug are sniffed and rise immediately to the brain.

Myself—AIDS & LIFE

I declared that I would not deteriorate and die. I am convinced that the Christian Science treatments given to me and that I gave myself helped make me strong—made me a conqueror over this dis-ease, AIDS.

After returning to the States and seeing the condition of Larry and other individuals with AIDS, I knew that I was winning the battle. I made a strong affirmation to myself that I would never let myself get into that extremely debilitated state and would do all I could to keep myself well—physically, mentally, and spiritually.

From the time the doctors came in and told me that they were going to do the AIDS antibody test, I immediately, in my mind, knew that I would test positive to the disease. I kept telling myself even back then that I refused to accept this dis-ease in my body. I've yet to let down my defenses against this dis-ease and I don't plan to ever do so.

I consider my body to be my Temple in which I house my three-part being: body, mind, and spirit. If I don't have control over my body, then who, pray tell, does?

Emotional States

Emotional states need to be monitored and either openly expressed or otherwise worked out.

Depression lowers the immune system. There's no question about it.

Hope is considered to be a good quality, but I don't have hope. To me, to have hope of something means you don't have it and are expecting a "magic solution." Hope implies doubt.

The only "Fear" I could say I have (and it's not really fear) is that I don't want to ever see myself lying in bed so incapacitated that I must have people waiting on me, with my senses and brain no longer in contact. That's what happened to my lover; he suffered so very much, and his mind left him three months before his death. I was there at all times to care for his needs. I don't want to see that happen to me, yet I would again care for someone else if he were in that condition.

The only time I find myself getting slightly ill, (I don't want to say "sick" because I haven't been sick for so long now), is when I get depressed, and yet there is no need for me to get depressed. I have so many supportive, true friends and family and I'm active in many projects and volunteer work, that depression shouldn't even exist for me.

Working in a very busy Emergency Room, I take care of many AIDS patients. I thoroughly love my job and it helps keep me on an even keel in my life. But at the present time I am thinking of Larry, my partner who died two years ago, his mother who died almost to the day one year ago, and my own father who passed away three years ago this month....So I'm dealing with a very heavy "death-memory" at present. But it shouldn't be a time for depression, because I feel that the departed are very happy now and in the spirit state and I should be happy for them and release them from earthly bonds to help them expand in their spiritual world.

My Spiritual Life and Meditation

One needs to separate a religious life from spiritual life. Religious life is, e.g., what the Catholic church teaches is right or wrong. I no longer follow its doctrines. But in spiritual life, I can make contact within myself to that level which is always awake, but which we as mortals are not always aware of.

I strongly believe in meditation. I think everyone should do it, even if he/she doesn't understand what it is. Meditation is basically relaxing the body, getting rid of ALL thoughts that enter one's mind. You may concentrate on a certain word or sound that has no meaning to you, such as "Om." You could pick up a basic meditation book or one of

Louise Hay's tapes or just lie back and relax; if you can't get into the train of thought needed, don't get discouraged. In time, and when your subconscious is ready, it will all fall into place, but don't stop trying. Remember to always keep blocking your mind from all the interference that will try to enter, such as "did I remember to?"... or "what am I going to do about...?" or "well, I guess this isn't working."...Just continue to block, block, and block and listen to the voice on the tape or be ready to hear the voice that is within you. This type of relaxation is very good for the inner self and for healing.

There are many persons who feel that if they can't see something with the eyes or touch it with the hands, then they can't believe in it. To these persons, I ask, "Do you believe in God?" and when they answer "Of course I do," I then ask them to show Him to me. "You can't show me God and yet you believe in Him." So I ask you to give these powers, this energy force that's all around us and your inner self (spirit/soul) a chance, because they do exist and you will find much inner peace and happiness in meditation.

"He advances most in divine Science who meditates most on infinite spiritual substance and intelligence," wrote Mary Baker Eddy.[3] And I study her works daily.

Accentuate the Positive!

AIDS proved to be an opportunity for me, with fantastic growth mentally, psychologically, and spiritually.

In the beginning, thoughts went through my mind such as: "Am I really going to die from this or can I change what medical science is saying?" Then I kept thinking: "What can I do" to help myself. I did much research, and still do, on syphilis/hepatitis B, drugs, stress, the immune system and everything else related to AIDS. I started creating my own hypothesis. For two years I've been saying that syphilis and hepatitis are somehow related to AIDS, and lo and behold, the medical researchers are now just realizing it. Many ideas that I strongly believe in through what I learned in my Western medicine training are being validated today.

I believe there's an inner spirit that's directing me. I get these insights and often I think I'm being told something that I should pay attention to.

My greatest strength has been and is my inner self (spirit). That's my guidance in keeping me well. A strictly positive approach to everything is required. It all has been a positive experience for me.

I kept telling myself that my illness was a temporary condition and that I was not going to die from it. That's the way I will continue to feel. I am helping others with these same concepts.

Drugs or "Naturals" to Cure Disease?

I don't know of any drug that will actually cure a disease. I feel that the body cures itself. We have been trying to find a "cure" for so many forms of cancer and yet nothing. Western medicine, as we know it, with its chemical drugs, is only a couple of hundred years old. People today should investigate herbal therapy. After all, didn't our ancestors and the Egyptians, American Indians, Chinese, and many other nations use herbs thousands of years ago for healing? And people should look into other natural therapies also.

I've watched cancer patients cure themselves with homeopathic therapies and other natural therapies, but not medical therapies. But we know the ways of the doctors. For them it's much easier to say, "Well, it's too bad but you're going to die within six months; everything has been done." Many patients won't accept this and that's basically how I was and still am.

I've heard many people saying: "My doctor told me I won't recover and that I should start preparing my will," etc....

What gives doctors the right to play God? Some doctors get even more specific and tell a patient that he has only three or four weeks left to live. Can you imagine what that does to these people emotionally? Poor advice like this (called "mental malpractice" in Christian Science) lowers the patient's immune system right away. Words are very powerful and we must choose and use them carefully. Doctors need to be re-educated, and this time in the power of the mind!

If we spread the holistic approach, I think we in the U.S. stand a strong chance of winning the battle over this spreading epidemic. We must get strong and prove to our government that the tax monies are being wasted in drug research, and are needed for education and teaching the public other therapies in caring for the sick.

Even basic things like hygiene and eating habits are important. Even the water you drink is important. Try spring water, or, if you have to, distilled water; it's far better than drinking the tap water with all its contaminants and chemicals. Some people feel that if the government agencies say that the water is OK for the public, then it is. But it is not OK and is not healthful, especially for someone who is sick. Remember that our bodies are composed of up to 75% water, so the water we use should be the best water available.

My Supplement Program

What products did I use in my program to overcome AIDS?

I have always been a firm believer in vitamins. At present, I'm on megadoses of various vitamins, especially vitamin C, taking over 45,000 mg. per day. My treatments consist of vitamin & herbs, EggsACT (an AL-721 workalike), aloe vera, chlorophyll and wheatgrass (for their oxygen properties), and I've even started experimenting with food grade hydrogen peroxide 35% solution which I read about in *Con-*

quering AIDS Now! I also drink a powder solution called Immunectar, by Nature's Plus, which is loaded with vitamins and herbs such as egg yolk lecithin, colostrum, CoQ10, Beta Carotene, SOMA and about 14 other ingredients. I've investigated, decided what was best for me, and made a total commitment.

Also, I belong to the support group described, keep the book, *Conquering AIDS Now!* as an AIDS guide, and continue with acupuncture. I started acupuncture not as an AIDS alternative treatment, but to deal with my deep depression over the loss of my lover. Losing Larry was so very difficult for me, but my spirit is once again on the rise.

My acupuncturist also has me on three different Chinese herbs: Compassionate Sage, Placenta and Quiet Contemplate. I know that one of these helps to cool down my body system, as I tend to be a very warm-blooded person. I've also visited an herbologist to decide on the best herbal program for me. He uses an aggressive/passive, masculine/feminine, type of theory. Through talking with you, he first decides into what classification to place you, and uses animals as examples, such as "are you more like a lion or more like a lamb?" He states that one doesn't need more than five different herbs. I have two bad addictions—nicotine and caffeine. Soon I hope to stop both (one at a time, though).

Education and Counseling Requirements

How can individuals protect themselves? Education, Education, and more Education.

If someone has been with a partner for perhaps several years, and there are problems in the relationship, I think the couple should get counseling or work on what is wrong with the relationship and should stay together. If one is going out to a singles bar, whether heterosexual or homosexual, to meet someone new, I think he should date this person for awhile and get to know him or her and a little of their past for the last five or six years. If there is feeling there and one wants to get together more intimately, he should be honest and admit to the other person that he is positive to the virus, and see that the other person understands the risks. But take precautions. Then, I think, they should go ahead, because after all, we are human, we do have feelings and emotions, and one can't deprive himself of sex forever, unless he chooses to remain celibate.

"Safe Sex"

I don't believe that "safe sex" is really safe—unless one limits his sex to mutual masturbation or engages in lovemaking, which to me is from the waist up, and that includes kissing/touching. These things might qualify as "safe sex", but anything below the waist, such as anal intercourse even with so-called protection, I call that "unsafe sex." I don't personally believe that the AIDS virus is spread through oral sex. The reason I say this is because (1) the virus dies seconds after exposure to air (which is always flowing in and out of your mouth), (2) the hydrochloric acid constantly being excreted kills the virus and finally, (3) the combined acids in the stomach make it impossible for this virus to survive. So all that is being absorbed into the body system is the dead virus, I believe.

As far as the Masters & Johnson's study that says the virus definitely exist in the saliva, I would like to see positive proof. I don't believe anything they have put out in their book and I hope that some of our researchers, scientists, and Surgeon General Koop come through and prove that they are wrong. Masters & Johnson are going to make a fortune on their book, *Crisis: Heterosexual Behavior/AIDS*. Some people will make the mistake of buying it, but waste their money. These authors are adding more panic to an already panic-stricken heterosexual society and I don't feel that this is fair to the public.

Virus Reinfection

It's difficult to confirm that people are reinfected by the virus. I think that if you're with a lover in a long-term relationship and you are both infected, then only one strain of the virus has been passed between the two of you. Yet if you go out and engage in multiple sex relationships, it is possible to pick up different strains of the virus, so I suppose one can be reinfected.

About Blood Transfusions

I am not convinced that the blood today is safe. The reason I say this is: a person could be tested for the virus today and he is negative. He gives a pint of what he thinks is good blood, and three months from now he either shows HIV antibodies or has AIDS. The antibodies didn't show up in the original testing, yet the virus was present and the blood that has been transfused into someone else's body may be carrying the virus and that person may get the disease.

Holistic healing and alternative therapies are inexpensive, are shown to enhance the immune system and will probably be front runners in the cure. But the government, scientists and manufacturers aren't going to make any profit on them—hence the lack of publicity and utilization.

Diagnosis and Misdiagnosis

I am firmly convinced that many people are misdiagnosed and I do believe that Western medicine tends to put people on the wrong track of treatment. Also, it puts fear into an individual who may be negative but shows a false positive. He's so full of fear that he has placed himself/herself at risk. Yes, Fear will lower the immune system.

Kindness in Nurses is Vital (Life-Giving)

In the medical profession, I meet the most belligerent and cold-hearted doctors and nurses. They don't seem to understand or don't want to, or they have a blocked mind to this dis-ease. I've seen this time and time again, from hospital to hospital, and it's really a pity. These are "educated" people and should have more open minds. They are in a healing profession, and should be kind.

"An ill-tempered, complaining, or deceitful person should not be a nurse. The nurse should be cheerful, orderly, punctual, patient, full of faith—receptive to Truth and Love."[4]

My Friendships

My friends have helped me tremendously. There is no question about it. They are great. I keep thinking of the song "That's What Friends Are For." About 90% of the friends I have now are new. After returning from Cairo, many of my old friends had died and now the friends I am making, mostly HIV positive/AIDS people, are true, sincere, caring friends and I am lucky to have them.

It's really amazing. There are friends I went to high school with 25 years ago. I told a couple of them about my sickness because a class reunion was coming up. I've had calls from five or six from the class. Some said, "Please be at the reunion; you have our support. If you have to come home to stay, we're here to take care of you." You don't know how that made me feel. Here are people I haven't seen in 25 years giving me such support; it was really rewarding to me.

I have lost eighteen personal friends to this dis-ease, but I have not lost any of my newly-acquired friends who are either HIV-Positive or have AIDS. I have made beautiful new friends through "Positive Immunity" and other AIDS groups.

Who Helped Me Most

My life really changed since I got involved with my acupuncturist, with Ellie Kierson and her excellent spiritual guidance, and the many other persons who are involved in alternative treatments. I think *Conquering AIDS Now!* by Gregory and Leonardo is one of the best books published on AIDS and believe me, I have read many and have done more research than most doctors on this dis-ease, AIDS.

My R.N.-Christian Science friend in Saudi Arabia helped me a great deal, teaching me that we must rebuke disease, lift our thoughts to higher spiritual levels, and learn about the power of Spirit.

My Plans for the Future

I have no long-range plans. I like living just one day at a time. I wake up each day, glad to be here, happy to be healthy. I plan on being around for a long time and I do want to do more travelling. I would very much like to return to Cairo, Egypt and make my home there, as that is one place in the world where I felt that I really fit in. Much love, simplicity and purity are expressed in that country, I found. At present my plans are to continue to help those who are less fortunate than I am right now with this dis-ease. I try to get them on a road of permanent recovery through my volunteer work—30 hours per week.

AIDS and the Media

I don't believe anything I read or hear through the media on AIDS unless it comes directly from the CDC in Atlanta, Georgia, or *USA Today,* a newspaper with excellent coverage on AIDS. I do read, however, merely to see what the latest money-making gimmicks are, and I realize that the companies must sell newspapers and magazines. They ignore the fact there are survivors of this disease. If they say that AIDS is not a deadly disease, that's not going to sell papers. Our society thrives on morbid news. As long as the papers say "death rate up, new symptoms of AIDS, etc.", people grab the newspapers immediately.

Our paper here, *The Washington Post,* for years was very anti-homosexual and started out being anti-AIDS, but lately they have let up quite a bit. But still, when I read these articles, I laugh...you must if you are going to survive.

AIDS and Profits

Who is making the most money from AIDS?

Definitely not the insurance companies, but for certain the doctors, the hospitals, and the pharmaceutical companies.

The insurance companies own many of the HMO's (health maintenance organizations). They own the hospitals and tell the doctors what procedures they must use. So they are becoming a monopoly on medical care.

The biggest profits are being made by the drug companies. They keep coming out with new drugs. Now it's Amphilgen, which is supposed to be better than AZT. The advantage of Amphilgen is that it has fewer, if any, side effects and blood transfusions aren't needed. Ya! Why don't they try investing some of this money into natural therapies and find out where the answer really is? At present the Amphilgen study is being done at The George Washington University in Washington, D.C., the National Institute of Health, in Bethesda, MD. (suburb of D.C.) and a few hospitals on the West coast. But once again I say: It doesn't cure you; it only helps to extend your life, and what kind of life will that be? I speak from experience.

Abbott, the company that formulated the AIDS test, took in $3.1 billion in its first year's sales, with a profit of $646.1 million.

This disease has caused many corporations to make megabucks and will keep making megabucks. The government subsidy of AIDS "research and development" is rapidly approaching the trillion-dollar figure!

I feel that the cure is in the air, but the manufacturers risk to lose billions. AZT, for example, is bringing in up to $1,000 or more per person per month. This dis-ease is a money-making proposition.

How Many People With AIDS?

Many more people have this disease than we know. There's no question about it. I learn of at least two or three old friends every week who have been keeping it under, coming out and asking me, "I got it, what should I do?"

Perhaps one-eighth of the population has AIDS now, in my opinion. Of course, there is a lot of misdiagnosis right now. For example, and this is true: someone comes into our Emergency Room who is a known IV drug user, or gay, who has some of the classic symptoms (fever, night sweats, diarrhea, weight loss, etc.), and right away the diagnosis on his chart is "AIDS." This is very bad, especially when the individual's insurance company gets the bill. Here we have the doctor putting down "AIDS, HIV POSITIVE" and we don't even know for sure. We ask the patient "have you been tested for the AIDS virus?" "No." Yet the doctors are putting down "HIV POSITIVE". This is being done at one of the largest hospitals in Washington, D.C. that handles most of the AIDS patients.

One wonders how they can do that. I'm sure that insurance companies are having a field day with cancellations and raising premiums. Also, I'm seeing an increasing number of women coming in. We have a large black population in the Washington area and I'm seeing many black heterosexual females who are either IV drug users, or who have had or have bisexual boyfriends or straight boyfriends who are IV drug users. Of course, I can't say that they have AIDS because most of them haven't been tested, but many of them say they have been tested and are positive. But most of the false diagnoses of AIDS on the charts are being done by the doctors.

My Advice to Persons With AIDS

I feel that every individual who is diagnosed as HIV positive, as having ARC or AIDS, can also get well. First, I feel they should stop the antibiotics, the IV pentamadine, and especially AZT. Let these individuals turn to Holistic Healing and yet keep their doctors for times of extreme need when a little help from medicine may help—for example, medication for pain relief. I really feel in my heart that this illness can be beaten, but our doctors and our hospitals are not yet open to the holistic side of healing. Our society has been brainwashed into Western medicine with all its chemical drugs. Western medicine as we know it is only a couple of hundred years old. But I ask you—how many years have the Chinese been using acupuncture and herbs successfully? <u>Over two thousand five hundred years!</u>

What Worked for Me Can Work For You

Regardless of what the illness is, whether it's something that's life threatening or mild, I feel that my methods can work for everyone. Regardless of what your religious beliefs are, even if you're an atheist, if you can learn just a little about Holistic Healing, a little about nutrition and a little about meditation, then you're on the road to progress. You start your work from there. Once the new thoughts are impregnated into the brain, then they're transferred to your subconscious mind and you'll be open to suggestions. It's getting that thought into the brain that is the toughest part. I am convinced it will work for anyone and everyone and this includes young people also, because children have very good imaginations and they can be taught meditation or/and visualization with little difficulty.

Drugs and Side Effects

My doctor is pushing me to take AZT and Acyclovir in combination, but I have emphatically refused and told my doctor that there are side effects from both drugs. If I am feeling great and have no more signs and symptoms, why should I take a drug that might harm my health?

As an AIDS volunteer, I counsel many individuals and encourage them to consider other ways of healing besides experimental drugs that can have harmful side effects. If the drugs that are used for AIDS were not harmful, they would not be listed in the Physicians Desk Reference (PDR) and a prescription for their use would not be necessary. All synthetic and chemical drugs can have side effects.

Individuals should be told of the side effects of drugs. For example, Pentamadine, used to treat lung infections, often has side effects, one of which is hypotension (that could lead to cardiac arrest).

Side effects of AZT and Bactrim are too numerous to mention. So, if the patient elects to use drugs, he must be monitored closely and taken off the drug if side effects occur.

Symptoms and Diagnosis

Concerning treatment of pneumocystis: patients should be informed that the diagnostic procedures can be inaccurate or dangerous. Sputum samples from the lungs are often difficult to obtain and tend to be inaccurate. A second diagnostic method is a biopsy which is a surgical procedure. It, however, must find the specific site of the infection to be accurate. An X-ray will show a clouded area, but does not necessarily show that it is the pneumocystis pneumonia. The bronchoscopy, the most definitive diagnostic tool yet, can be a dangerous procedure. It is a major surgery which requires anesthesia. Vocal cords can be injured. I know of a case where a man lost his voice, permanently, after a bronchoscopy.

I believe that if you look hard enough for something you will find it, even if it is not there. With a positive HIV test, the Merck Manual and the doctors' consensus of signs and symptoms determine if the disease is present. If an individual has the diagnosis of AIDS or pre-AIDS or is HIV positive, then certain symptoms have to be present. If they are not, medical science will look until they find them. And the patient, in wanting to cooperate with his doctor, will search and search until he finds the symptoms. If the mind can manifest burns under hypnosis, it surely can manifest symptoms such as AIDS.

Also, unresolved guilt from a destructive lifestyle can be channeled or redirected verbally to your doctor. Now both you and your doctor focus and solidify the belief that "if you've been naughty, you'll have to pay the price." Unresolved guilts often become expressed as physical symptoms.

A good physician should offer encouragement and support. Negative input is not beneficial to a patient. Generally, when one goes to a doctor he is in a physically and mentally weakened state. Therefore, to reinforce the idea that you are genetically weak or prone to AIDS/ARC/cancer, etc., not only makes you vulnerable, but sets the stage for disease because, after all, "doctors know best."

Be selective when you choose your doctor.

Most Important

The most important thing for a Person With AIDS to hear is that AIDS IS NOT A DEATH SENTENCE. Accept AIDS as a *learning experience to love.* Listen to what holistic medicine and alternative treatment have to offer you. Don't reject something just because you don't quite understand it. TRY IT! I have told this to many a person and it has helped.

QUESTION YOUR DOCTOR. Don't always accept his word. Ask him: "Why are you putting me on this and what are the side effects, the benefits, and what has been proven with this drug?" Really get after him. DON'T LET HIM START DIRECTING YOUR LIFE, AND I STATE AGAIN "IT'S YOUR LIFE, NOT HIS."

*   *   *   *   *

If the reader wants to contact Jeffrey Migota, write the publisher, Tree of Life Publications. He wants to help Persons With AIDS—from his standpoint of love, compassion, and knowledge. As he previously stated,
"That's what friends are for."

WHAT JEFFREY MIGOTA DID

• Being a nurse, he is familiar with medical procedures. Being a thinker[5], he sees through the belief that a patient can be drugged into health and that drugs cure disease. He knows about the side effects of all drugs.

• He was in Saudi Arabia at the time, where treatments are more primitive and where "high tech" medicine is not available. He found later this to be his protection, as all or most of the early Persons With AIDS died under Western medical treatment.

• He conveyed to his doctors the mode of treatment that he wanted, in Saudi Arabia. Upon returning to the U.S., he sought out alternative, natural therapies and spiritual paths.

• He saw his lover die after U.S. medical treatment, and did not want to experience the pain and suffering that Larry had gone through—all for naught.

• He saw the unreliability of the AIDS testing. Although the medical people advise patients that the tests are reliable, actually the results include false positives and false negatives.

• Much reading and introspection were part of his path. He found the spiritual writings of Mary Baker Eddy, and still studies, daily, a portion of her book, *Science and Health with Key to the Scriptures.*

• He also discovered the book *Conquering AIDS Now! Alternative, Natural Therapies,* by Gregory and Leonardo. Both books opened his eyes to ways of healing other than medical. He learned systematic undereating and adopted an almost vegetarian diet.

• He became involved with a self-healing group in Washington, D.C. called "People *Living* with AIDS." Weekly speakers address the issue of AIDS and enlighten the members on various holistic healing modalities.

• One of the lecturers took a personal interest in him and shared his knowledge of therapies such as: the laying on of hands and other spiritual methods of healing; Reiki therapy (healing with energy fields); healing herbs, acupuncture, meditation, visualizations, affirmations, etc.

• He had an inward conviction that he could heal himself. He believed in himself and had a very high self-esteem.

• He learned how to meditate and how to feel an inward calm. This ability helped him in stressful situations at the hospital.

• He was thoughtful and caring for others during his sickness.

• After the symptoms diminished, he immediately started educating others on what he had learned. He enjoys sharing and helping others.

• He refused to allow any negative input to interfere with or postpone his healing.

• He stayed away from negative people and made many new positive friends.

• Under the natural and spiritual regimes of his own choosing he recovered quickly.

• Jeffrey Migota's messages to all those affected by this dis-ease AIDS are: NEVER GIVE UP! And: please have peace with yourself. Don't strive, but thrive on being happy. Love yourself and all others. Peace, love and health be with you.

NOTE:
Jeffrey recommends this book: *Superimmunity*, by Paul Pearsall, and remarks on the import of this quotation from the book: "If AIDS teaches us anything, it teaches us that a holistic approach will be the only answer for the ultimate survival of our civilization." (Page 222.)[6]

---

[1]   Eddy, Mary Baker. "Unity of Good", page 9, in *Prose Works*. The Christian Science Publishing Society, Boston, MA.
[2]   Gregory, Scott and Leonardo, Bianca. *Conquering AIDS Now!* Tree of Life Publications, 1986; Warner Books, 1987. (Pages 93-94 in Warner Books edition.) Also see book *Cancer & Other Diseases Caused by Meat Consumption—Here's the Evidence*, by Bianca Leonardo.
[3]   Eddy, Mary Baker. *Miscellaneous Writings*, page 309. The Christian Science Publishing Society, Boston, MA.
[4]   Eddy, Mary Baker. *Science and Health with Key to the Scriptures*, page 395.
[5]   Eddy, Mary Baker. "The time for thinkers has come." Page vii, in *Science and Health with Key to the Scriptures* .
[6]   Pearsall, Paul. *Superimmunity* . Los Angeles: J. P. Tarcher, 1987.

PEOPLE LIVING WITH AIDS—
A Self-healing Group

This support group is facilitated by Ellie Kierson and promotes self-healing through on-going sessions. The group draws together to provide love and support to each person, to empower each person to take control of his health and his life, and to provide him with the experience, knowledge, information and skills to empower his body to heal itself.

These sessions are totally inter-active and participatory and offer:

- Sharing and individual attention
- Much deeper understanding of the mind-body-spirit connection
- Time for and teaching of meditation and relaxation techniques
- Supporting and nurturing a Positive Attitude (Attitudinal Healing)
- The opportunity to get to the cause of the dis-ease in one's life and to transform it
- Being introduced to and learning various Self-Healing techniques
- Participation in and presentation of Traditional/Alternative/Holistic Medicines (i.e.: Western Medicine, Chinese Medicine, Chiropractic, Crystals, Massage, Music, Colors, Homeopathy, etc.)
- Presenting many and varied methods, points of view and information about healing through videos/tapes/speakers
- Supporting each person in the development of his own healing programs
- Supporting each person in LIVING with and CONQUERING AIDS

PEOPLE LIVING WITH AIDS—A Self-Healing Group
Location: Riva Market Research, 4609 Willow Lane, Bethesda, MD.
Ellie Kierson, Director Phone: (301) 921-0091

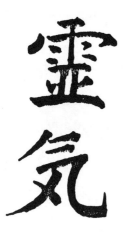

Reiki

"I did not arrive at my understanding of the fundamental laws of the universe through my rational mind."

—Albert Einstein

Einstein expressed a deep-seated inner feeling when he declared that light and matter are interchangeable. Explained in the formula $E=MC^2$, his landmark pronouncement actually appears to be a rediscovery of what mystics and others have known for many centuries: THE POINT OF LIGHT WITHIN. THE INNER FLAME. UNIVERSAL LIFE ENERGY.

Reiki (rei = universal, ki = vital life force) is a Japanese word representing Universal Life Energy, the energy which is all around us. Reiki, when activated and applied for purposes of healing, addresses body, mind, and spirit. It accelerates the body's ability to heal physical ailments and opens the mind and spirit to the causes of disease and pain, the necessity for taking responsibility for one's life and the joys of balanced wellness. The Usui System of Reiki is a natural healing art which uses Reiki in these ways.

This system was born out of the experience and dedication of Dr. Mikao Usui, a Japanese Christian educator who, in the 1800's, responded to a challenge from his university students by undertaking an extensive study of the healing phenomena of history's greatest spiritual leaders. Through travel, study, research and meditation, he evolved a healing system based on ancient Buddhist teachings written in Sanskrit. He spent the rest of his life practicing and teaching this method of natural healing, which involves attunement to the universal energy and the laying on of hands. The Usui System of Reiki continues to be taught by Reiki Masters who are trained in the original traditions of Reiki and whose personal and professional lives are committed to this healing art and the lifestyle which it engenders.

The technique is effective for prevention of diseases and energy imbalances on all levels of Being, as well as dealing with chronic or current issues. It can be used in conjunction with any other technique of health-care treatment as well as any other personal growth therapy. It does not conflict with traditional medicine, but can be used with it or as an additional source for restoring vital energy and promoting health and well-being.

A classic treatment consists of hands-on application of several positions beginning at the top of the head, and moving downward to the base of the spine. A full treatment takes from one and a half to two hours. The first steps involve applying one's hands to positions that cover the head and neck, and impact the eyes, sinus tracts, brain, pituitary and pineal glands, throat and thyroid gland. The next steps apply hands to the front of one's spleen, pancreas, intestines, bladder, and reproductive organs. The final steps apply one's hands to areas of the back, and involve the heart, lungs, adrenal glands, kidneys, spinal cord, lower back and intestines. Part of this treatment includes balancing and aligning the seven major chakras (or subtle centers of energy) from the base of the spine to the top of the head. In a session one's life force comes into balance and harmony with the Universal Energy, promoting healing and "wholing" from within our body-mind-spirit dynamics.

In my practice, I work with many people living with AIDS, who have chosen Reiki treatments as a complement to their entire healing program. These people report that during and for some time after sessions they become deeply relaxed—releasing and letting go totally of fear, anxiety and stress (all immune suppressors). They have a deep inner sense of peace and general well-being. Aches, pains and physical discomfort are alleviated. One's breathing becomes deep, even and easier. They experience a profound sense of balance and harmony—physically as well as emotionally, mentally and spiritually. There is an increase in one's energy level. Reiki seems to support the acceleration of the healing process (i.e., moving through colds very quickly, recovering from surgery at a much increased pace, mending of wounds, etc.) and supports the system in mobilizing all its inherent capacities to heal itself.

Over a period of time, people notice an increased sense of self-awareness and understanding, leading to balance, harmony and responsibility in all aspects of their lives.

Reiki is an excellent addition and complement to one's over-all program and should not replace the appropriate or proper health care.

GUIDED IMAGERY AND MUSIC (GIM)

This is a specific method developed by Helen Bonny. It is a method of Self-exploration in which classical music is used to access the imagination. It includes listening to classical music in a relaxed state, allowing the imagination to come to conscious awareness and sharing these awarenesses with a guide. The interaction among listener, music and guide is what makes GIM unique.

For thousands of years and throughout many cultures, the imagination has been regarded as a powerful agent in the healing process. Today many experimental and clinical studies have shown that imagery can help bring about rapid and far-reaching emotional, psychological, physiological and spiritual changes. Music is a powerful stimulant of the imagination, and research has shown that we tend to generate more imagery with a greater intensity and duration with music than without.

This combination of Imagery and Music in the GIM method has proven to be quite potent—with the potential for bringing about rapid change, growth, self-understanding, ordering of the psyche, integration, spiritual development and healing.

The process consists of a series of individual GIM sessions, conducted in a one-to-one relationship with a trained guide. More information regarding the specifics of the method (i.e., what happens in a session, how many sessions recommended, etc.) can be obtained from a GIM Facilitator.

In my practice, I have been and am working with many people living with AIDS who have chosen GIM as a complementary method in their healing programs. These people report that they come to an overall and general sense of well-being, peace, centeredness and calm. That stress, fear, anxiety, depression, anger, resentment and grief (negative emotional states that contribute to the suppression of the immune system) are completed and fade, and that a more positive stance and experience towards their life and living emerges. The past is released and healed—and the future discovered and opened up. PWAs discover within themselves a genuine sense of HOPE and purpose, strength and courage. They are able to come to terms with and transform their experience of the disease. They connect with their most inner and higher self-tapping profound and inherent potentials for change, growth and healing. They feel nurtured and empowered to make and act on choices and changes that are appropriate for their own health and well-being.

—Ellie B. Kierson
Guided Imagery and Music Facilitator

Roger Walther

Five years ago, Roger Walther was running a telephone "sexual fantasy service"[1], and was sexually compulsive. He had a promiscuous and destructive lifestyle, which resulted in AIDS-Related Complex, diagnosed by Dr. Michael Gottlieb of UCLA (May 1, 1984).

He tried suicide twice, but "didn't have the guts to do it." There was no suicide, but his life "stopped dead"—until he

---

[1] A telephone referral service from which homosexual men can obtain numbers of willing partners for the act of arousing the sexual state, although in absentia. It is a completely anonymous experience. The caller describes his sexual condition, and the salacious conversation begins. Verbal abuse sometimes heightens the pleasure of the resultant erection and orgasm.

totally changed his consciousness and lifestyle to one of spiritual thinking and growth, constructive activity, and habits of health. He is now 34, with the promise of a whole life to live. In his words:

"I had to learn to love myself and to take power in my life."

Roger Walther's Adventure

On days that I feel spiritual, I believe that AIDS is caused by a mental state, specifically, a lack of self-love. When I am in more of a physical consciousness, which is most of the time, I feel that AIDS has physical causes and attacks those who are open to the disease. There are such factors as many antibiotics, other drugs, a poor diet. Gay men are especially prone to eating lots of sweets and have a generally poor diet. Also, I believe the disease is spread primarily through sexual contact. If one is in good shape physically, he can resist any virus. No matter how it penetrates the body, the immune system should be able to handle it, I believe.

To summarize this point: I believe the co-factors in the gay community causing them to get AIDS are: recreational and doctor-given drugs; poor nutrition; insufficient rest and sleep, and over-use of sex. Numerous orgasms per day deplete the body of minerals, other essential vitamins, proteins, and amino acids—plus the life force energy.

I was extremely promiscuous. I've had gonorrhea about twenty times in my life and syphilis at least three times. Large quantities of antibiotics were pumped into my body to treat these diseases, as well as other ailments. I believe that all these antibiotics caused the candidiasis[1] from which I now suffer. I also had hepatitis A and B.[2] The doctors used penicillin and tetracyline to treat these conditions. These drugs were so aggravating to my liver, I could not tolerate it. I had such a high antibody titer (serum blood level) that the doctors used it make a hepatitis vaccine for others. So my serum was used for vaccines every week, and I got paid for it.

Approximately eight months later, I started showing symptoms of AIDS. Many people may have become infected from my blood, but I didn't know I had AIDS, and the doctors didn't know it. If I had had any clue or suspicion, I would have stopped giving my blood.

As for recreational drugs, I took LSD about fifteen times, and smoked marijuana bi-weekly for several years. I stopped before I got sick.

I visited my family in Peoria, Illinois for the holidays in 1985. On December 26, I went to the hospital there. They diagnosed me as having AIDS. I was admitted and the doctors

---

[1] Candida albicans is a fungus overgrowth, resulting in candidiasis, which depresses the immune function and leads to a myriad of health problems. These could be allergies, intestinal malfunction, and possible cancer and birth defects. The brain is affected, and memory loss, mood swings, inability to concentrate, depression, anxiety, and frustration are some of the manifestations. The senses can also show undesirable changes. Tens of millions of Americans suffer from it, possibly one in three persons, and most Persons With AIDS.

Causes are antibiotics, oral contraceptives, and fermented foods such as alcohol and cheese; also sugar and other refined carbohydrates.

[2] Hepatitis A: spread primarily by fecal-oral contact, through blood and possibly secretions that are infectious. Water and food-borne epidemics are common. Ingestion of raw, contaminated shellfish can be responsible.

Hepatitis B: transmitted by contaminated blood or needles; sharing of needles by drug abusers often responsible.

Both can be spread sexually.

put me on oxygen the minute I got into the hospital. I had difficulty breathing; I was blue and I was blacking out. While in isolation, I was treated with Bactrim intravenously. I experienced bad reactions: skin rashes and fevers. My reactions were so extreme that I had to be taken off Bactrim. They did a lung biopsy. The air passages closed and I had to be intubated. This is a procedure where a tube is forced down one's throat toward the lungs, forcing oxygen into the lungs. It is an emergency procedure. I was released from the hospital, but having AIDS frightened me; I knew I had to make some changes in my lifestyle, which I did. The changes were gradual; my consciousness had to change first. It was an evolutionary process.

I feel I have totally recovered from the disease, and my life is so much more peaceful. What I am doing with my life is very different now, and I don't feel the fear and the stress I had before.

As for sex, I'm not having any. I learned Tibetan methods for pulling the sexual energy to the higher chakras. Through a healer, I experienced chakra balancing. Then I got a book from a friend on Tibetan exercises, commonly called The Five Rites. The book is entitled *Ancient Secret of the Fountain of Youth* and is about chakra balancing.[1] I listened to tapes on chakra meditations, and these have been pivotal. According to Chinese medicine, every time a man ejaculates, he loses Yuan Chi energy.

(Could the answer lie here—for persons with great and seemingly uncontrollable sexual drives?—Authors.)

It was my choice to raise my sexual energies rather than continue with the promiscuous lifestyle. At this time, there is no one I want sex with, but I'm always open to meet someone.

---

[1] See section on Rites at end of this chapter.

On the subject of self-esteem: before the disease, I thought of myself as an odd mixture of a terrific, intellectual human being, but also a nasty S.O.B..

I had attempted suicide twice in my life before the diagnosis, and seriously considered it after the onset of the disease—before the big shift.

What form of suicide was I contemplating? I would go swimming in the pool and try to stay down. After a dive, I hoped I would not come up, but the force of the water always brought me to the surface. I did not have the guts to try another way.

Now my attitude has changed dramatically. I love myself. I would like to love myself more. Suicide is not a choice for me now; life is. I'm learning to love others and not be so judgmental. I open my heart; I am a much nicer, more gentle human being.

I was an unwanted child; my mother had wanted to abort me, and I was told about it. This caused me to feel much anger toward my parents, but I have now released that. My parents are still alive, and I see them.

(Shortly after the interview that is the basis of this chapter, Roger left Los Angeles and returned to Peoria, Illinois, to live with his parents. See the end of chapter for the dramatic change in this relationship.)

Since my bout with pneumocystis, I don't feel vulnerable to this disease any more. I rarely have a cold. Of course, I produced the former stress, so it is a matter of controlling my life.

I wish I had known three years ago, what I know about AIDS now. I feel I have my candidiasis under control. My lack of self-love and a heavy sugar intake were factors in this condition. I was a pig with cookies and ice cream!

Being sick has done for me exactly what I wanted to have happen in my life. It gave me a choice—to either live or die. Dying was my first choice. I had gotten so close to dying. But somehow, somewhere, I changed the thought. The illness gave me the opportunity to grow, and grow, and grow. Daily, I found myself becoming a better human being. I let my past go; I released all negative memories, regrets, resentments, and became more willing and able to love others.

As for my friendships during the illness, they ran the whole gamut. I had a very close friend who couldn't deal with my sickness, could not tolerate being around me. My dearest friend has been incredibly loyal, calling me every week, day and night. My good friend and business partner went through major changes. The relationship has fallen apart, and we keep in contact, but the shift in my consciousness has alienated him. He also talks to me in an odd tone of voice, like this:

"How ARE you?" It's a disbelief that I am still alive.

"Are you still WELL?" There is fear in his voice. But new people I meet are delighted that I have overcome AIDS.

There is often some quite wonderful support. I find people who are willing to open their hearts to me. People are very beautiful and very giving. But the range is so great, it is dramatic.

The greatest shift in my thinking has been my spiritual growth. I was an atheist for nineteen years. Since AIDS, I pray daily, at least several times a day.

I have gone into rebirthing. This is a new breathing process, a technique that allows one to release the past and reprogram new thoughts. I consult my higher self now. I do channeling. This means to communicate with some entity who is totally in the spiritual realm. This consciousness speaks through certain individuals either departed or still on earth. Sai Baba is such a one—a highly developed, spiritual being in India.

I believe I would be completely well if I could totally surrender to God. In such a consciousness, there is trust in God; divine wisdom guides and protects you. This power has been so very good to me; this is why I am alive today. I am grateful, thankful. My aim is to feel and express that thankfulness and gratitude daily, hourly. This is practicing the presence of God, as Brother Lawrence called it, long ago.

What else started me on the new path? The AIDS Project Los Angeles was very helpful to my spiritual growth. The counselors said to me: "We want you to live; keep up your hope." They referred me to a book entitled *Getting Well Again* by Stephanie Matthews-Simonton and Dr. O. Carl Simonton. This was my first introduction to self-healing. I also came into contact with other books, people, and methods that teach using the mind for self-healing.

I attended monthly AIDS Update seminars called "Being Gay, Being Well." Individuals also inspired me. In this group, I met Louie Nassaney, who encouraged me to know that I could overcome the disease. I saw a flyer called "For Persons with AIDS and ARC" which gave me valuable information. One thing leads to another; it's like a chain.

By reading the book *The Anatomy of an Illness* by Norman Cousins[1], I learned about laughter as therapy.

I started doing aerobics and meditation. I learned to make a shift from left brain thinking to right brain thinking. The left brain is very analytical, and that is where I had lived most of my life. The right brain is receptive to God, and to

---

[1] Norman Cousins is also author of *The Healing Heart—Antidotes to Panic,* and creator of a video tape *The Healing Force.*

In 1964, former Saturday Review editor Norman Cousins contracted a rare, deadly disease. Refusing conventional treatment, he substituted positive thinking, humor, vitamin C and a powerful will to live. Making a remarkable complete recovery, he later suffered a debilitating heart attack, from which he again rehabilitated himself. Examining the potential of the individual's self-healing abilities, *The Healing Force* offers an in-depth discussion of Cousins' revolutionary approach to overcoming illness.

channel there is an element of surrender. So the spiritual side of you is the right brain working, and that is what mankind needs to develop.

I listened to a tape called "Self-Healing, Creating Your Health"—perhaps one thousand times! It suggests that you forgive your parents, and teaches creative visualization. I became involved in really reprogramming my mind, on the subconscious as well as the conscious level.

A series of tapes called "Maximum Immunity" is, I think, the best for reprogramming your mental attitudes to produce a healthier "you." (Available from the John David Learning Institute, Carlsbad, California.) *A Course in Miracles** also helped me. These volumes include a workbook for students and a manual for teachers, and there is group work.

Scott J. Gregory, co-author of *CONQUERING AIDS NOW!*, was supportive in my healing process. He advised me about diet and supplements, and also counseled me regarding how to view the disease, how to rid myself of the fear, panic, and conviction that AIDS was to be my cause of death, and soon. We both lived in Santa Monica. He often visited me—not as a paid professional, but as a friend.

What did I learn from my experience? I had to learn to love myself. I had to learn to change, to take charge of my life. I learned I am responsible for everything that happens in my life and every thought I think results in something happening "out there" in the world.

What do I think of "safe sex"? Masturbating is safe. Condoms are safe as long as they don't break. Spermicides are safe. Oral sex is highly dubious.

How can individuals protect themselves from AIDS? By changing their eating habits, reducing stress, stopping drugs, doing some exercise, developing some kind of spiritual

---

* See Bibliography.

endeavor and becoming involved in a therapy or work that enables them to love themselves more. Physical and sexual habits need to be altered.

A weakness—whether it be physical or mental—is what causes a breakdown of the body. It becomes subject to invading organisms. A shift in consciousness made me well.

What made me feel worse during the process? I felt worse when I didn't love myself, and when I felt alone, lonely, separated, and isolated, with a feeling that no one cared and that I was odd and different.

How did I get well? I opened my heart to God.

*   *   *   *   *

Roger Walther has had a great deal of personal growth in three years. It all started with the onset of AIDS, so the disease has been a blessing, after all. There is a phrase that says mankind chooses "suffering or Science (wisdom)." How one wishes that youngsters were instructed in these New Age disciplines (and some old-fashioned virtues, also), in order to spare them the years of wandering in false paths, wasted years, sickness, and sometimes early death.

Roger's friends have seen the remarkable difference in his personality; so have his parents. Before, there was a great alienation. Now, he and his parents are good friends. They enjoy their relationships.

One important thing he has learned from this disease is acceptance. He accepts the way people are and loves them, regardless. What would have irritated him before, he now laughs at.

He has changed his mother's diet to a more healthful one. She had arthritis and was always constipated. She's eating more grains and vegetables; the constipation is gone and the arthritis has lessened. Her health has markedly improved.

Before the great change in his consciousness, he was

always complaining. He was wrapped up in himself. Now he greets people with an enthusiastic "How are YOU?" He is very interested in other people.

He loves to laugh now. Taking a cue from Norman Cousins, who used laughter therapy for two serious illnesses, he watches funny old movies.

He says that humor is contagious, and has found that it helps relationships and works in all kinds of situations. He wants to share humor and the knowledge of its power with others. He is developing processes that teach people to laugh at those things in their lives which earlier caused anger, pain, or annoyance.

He will share these processes in a book called *Lighten Up!* He is currently writing a series of biographical sketches and humorous essays called "Laughing in the Face of Death."

Here is a remarkable case of a man who healed himself of AIDS, using natural and spiritual methods.

HERE IS HOLISTIC HEALING ("holistic" from the word "whole"). It covers all the aspects of man—BODY, MIND, AND SPIRIT.

In life stories such as these, we find hope in the surrounding gloom—for the dawning of a New Age.

WHAT ROGER WALTHER DID

• He searched for and found alternative healing methods and used them.

• He discovered how to live in the now. "One day at a time."

• He stopped his destructive lifestyle.

• He took responsibility for his health and his life.

• He didn't believe everything he read about AIDS and disease in general, presented in the media.

• He sought out those individuals who had conquered AIDS, and imitated their success.

• He did much reading on total health and on spiritual subjects.

• He learned to forgive and used practical techniques to release anger: rebirthing, affirmations, and turning to God. He asked those individuals whom he had hurt in the past to forgive him. And he forgave those who had hurt him, including his parents.

• He renewed his relationship with his family.

• He discovered natural healing and shared it with other persons, including his family.

• He found the book CONQUERING AIDS NOW! by Gregory and Leonardo, and it changed his life. Private counseling with Dr. Scott Gregory reframed his ideas about sickness and health, and he became able to cope with the fear and do something about it. Dr. Gregory helped him during the process of transformation.

• He worked on the spiritual, emotional, and psychological aspects of himself. Relatives, friends, and the authors saw the great change in him.

• He evolved from a critical, difficult, unhappy person into one who was happy, loving, and fun to be with.

• He became devoted to getting himself well and helping others.

• He sought that Power higher than ourselves, found it, and expressed it.

• He learned that much red meat aroused a sexual imbalance in his body. This realization was new to him.

• He established a balanced diet with limited animal protein. This made him more attuned, in touch, less aggressive. He conquered his negative emotional states. Balance was essential for him.

• He found that doctors know little about AIDS. He realized that his body could heal itself. He let it do so. But he gave it help—love and natural, gentle assistance.

• He used two important health regimes successfully: ancient Tibetan rejuvenation exercises called "The Five Rites," and rebirthing.

• Most individuals panic when they get seriously sick. He did not. He trusted his body to restore health to itself.

• Although once he had attempted suicide, Roger Walther has now learned to love life.

Postscript: Just before this book went to press, Roger wrote us, saying: "Leonard Orr, the man who discovered rebirthing, has invited me to do a metaphysical healing using the five elements: earth, air, water, fire, and mind.

"I am happy and positive and off any Western medicine. I recommend *A Course in Miracles*. God is with me and my consciousness is high. I am learning to love myself and others unconditionally. After my three months' training in advanced rebirthing, I hope to work at some holy place. I am letting God guide me."

—Roger Walther

THE ANCIENT TIBETAN RITES—
"FOUNTAIN OF YOUTH"

Roger Walther is using the "Ancient Tibetan Rejuvenation Rites" described in this book: *Ancient Secret of the Fountain of Youth* by Peter Kelder. Published by Harbor Press, P. O. Box 1656, Gig Harbor, WA 98335.

Do you dare to believe that in one month from now, as a result of the daily practice of five simple exercises that take about fifteen minutes a day, you can start feeling *dramatically* younger and stronger, you can triple your energy and feel all negativity draining, draining, draining, out of your mind?

That is what I feel is happening to me now after only three and a half weeks of practicing these "Ancient Tibetan Rejuvenation Rites." It's the most amazing and incredible thing I've ever experienced. From my own experience now, as well as from the testimonial letters in the book, I gather that what generally happens when you start doing these rites every day, is that for the first three weeks you wonder if they're really doing anything, and then the effects start hitting you!

The book contains the story of a British army colonel who was stationed in India in the 1920's. On several occasions he heard stories from the natives about a certain remote monastery in the Himalaya mountains in Tibet, where nobody grew old! Even persons well over 100 years of age retained the appearance and vigor of strong and healthy 25 to 35 year olds! Furthermore, old people who took up residence at the monastery began to look dramatically younger and stronger within a few months! (Was this the prototype for Shangri-La in "The Lost Horizon"—book by James Hilton and film?)

After the colonel retired, he found himself getting old and gray, and remembered these stories. He tried to persuade an American friend (the book's author), to accompany him to Tibet, where together they would search for the monastery with the Fountain of Youth. The friend was not thoroughly convinced that such a thing could be true and didn't want to take a chance. He thought it was an enormous amount of trouble—and a very long and expensive trip—for a possible wild goose chase. So the colonel took the trip alone to the Himalayas.

After months of searching, he found the monastery. There, he was immediately nicknamed "the Ancient One," because he looked so old. No one else looked old, although some claimed to be over 100 years of age.

The colonel began to follow the lifestyle and routine of the monastery. The lamas living there weren't trying to keep their knowledge secret, but the monastery was in such remote country, that they had very little contact with the world. Add to that the great skepticism and laziness of the human race, and one can see why the Rejuvenation Rites were a well-kept secret.

The lamas had a very healthy lifestyle in general, breathing the clean mountain air and working hard to grow their own food. This gave them exercise and pure, fresh, vegetarian food at the same time. They ate only one type of food at a meal usually, which helped them greatly to remain youthful and strong. But the colonel discovered that the core of their secret for staying young was five simple exercises, or rites, which they performed daily.

Within a few months, the colonel felt himself becoming completely transformed, dramatically stronger, and nobody called him "The Ancient One" any more.

One day he had the opportunity to look at himself in a mirror, which he had not been able to do for quite some time (the monastery not having any mirrors). He was amazed to see himself looking fifteen years younger! He stayed at the monastery for two years, then went to India to teach the rites to people there, then returned to America. He had become a very wise man. The book quotes him as saying: "So-called 'civilized' mankind is in truth living in the *darkest of dark ages!*"

When the colonel visited his American friend again, the man was unable to recognize him at first. The friend had expected a feeble 72-year-old, unable to walk without his cane. But the colonel looked like a strong and vigorous man in his early 40's! And, the author reports, the colonel continued to improve in the months that followed.

The colonel taught the rites to his friend, who immediately began practicing them and soon found himself benefitting wonderfully. They organized a class to teach the rites to others. All who practiced them diligently found themselves gaining astonishingly in youthful vitality within a few weeks. After a time the colonel continued on his travels, and his friend wrote this book. That was in the 1930's, and apparently the book became very rare, almost lost. In 1985 it was revived and published in a new edition by Harbor Press.

What are these rites, and how are they performed? They are simple to do, and the results are absolutely astonishing, amazing, and incredible. Try them; you have nothing to lose and benefits beyond your ability to imagine, to gain!

They have some resemblance to certain Yoga asanas, but are different and more powerful. As to how they work, the colonel explains in the book that they work on the seven major chakras. He says that the reason anyone gets old and enfeebled is that the spinning of these chakras gets "out of sync." Some chakras may get too slow, causing low energy in one area, others may get too fast, causing nervousness, and as a result of this lack of balance and harmony the body begins to decay. So the purpose of the rites is to get the chakras spinning again in proper synchronization with each other and at a speed appropriate to a strong and healthy 25 to 35-year-old—a person in the prime of life!

As a result of the sick and degenerate modern conditions of life as well as past karma and other influences, almost no one is in ideal health these days, so the rites are as beneficial to young people as the old.

They are helping me tremendously. In fact, I've never felt this good before, and I have been working on self-improvement quite intensively for fifteen years, trying at various times, hatha yoga, ajapa yoga, shabd-brahman yoga, kundalini maha yoga, karate, rebirthing, the raw food diet, re-evaluation counseling, dynamic meditation and Reichian therapy. I had been badly messed up and needed a lot of help, I admit it. All these therapies are fine, and they helped me. But I've *never* felt anything quite as good as these rites before, and they're not meant to replace anything else you are doing for physical fitness or enlightenment, but to supplement it and help make it work even better. So give these rites a try, please!

Regarding the practice of the rites: if you can't do one of the rites properly at first, don't be discouraged, just do the best you can. As in practicing hatha yoga or any other sort of physical exercise, your ability will gradually improve until you can do it properly. It is suggested that one practices the rites in the morning, doing in the first week three repetitions of each rite. Then, the second week, add two repetitions so you are doing five of each, then the next week, add two more, so you are doing seven, and so on , until you are doing 21 daily repetitions of each rite. Then, when you have been doing them for four months, if you would like to do them in the evening as well, start off again with three repetitions of each and gradually work up to 21 as before. About the third or fourth week of practice, you should feel and see remarkable results.

—Joe Alexander

Now, here are the rites, with sketches and instructions:

RITE NUMBER ONE

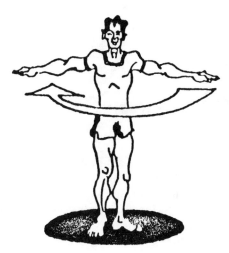

Stand with arms outstretched, horizontal to the floor, then spin around clockwise. (If a clock were lying face up on the floor, spin in the same direction the hands would move.) To keep from losing your balance, you can pick a point in front of you to focus on, then keep your eyes on it as long as you can as you begin spinning, then wrap your head around and return your focus to it as soon as possible.

RITE NUMBER TWO

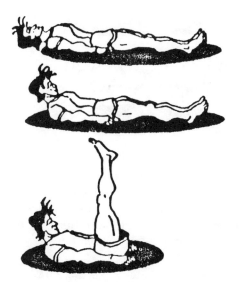

Lie on a mat on the floor with your arms extended at your sides, hands palms down, fingers together. Raise your head off the floor to touch chin to chest, lift your legs to vertical position, keeping the knees straight. Then slowly lower your head and legs to the floor and relax. Breathe in deeply as you lift your head and legs, out fully as you lower them, and maintain this rhythm of deep breathing between repetitions.

RITE NUMBER THREE

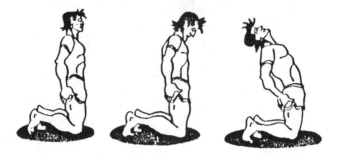

Kneel on a mat on the floor, body erect with hands against thigh muscles. Then incline your head forward to touch chin to chest, then throw your head and neck back as far as you can, breathing in deeply and leaning backward arching your back. Brace hands against thighs for support as you lean back. Then breathe out fully as you return to original position, maintaining this rhythm of deep breathing between repetitions.

RITE NUMBER FOUR

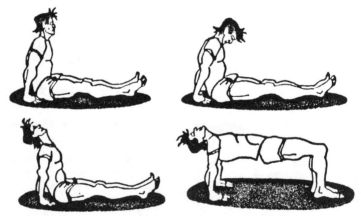

Sit on mat on floor, legs straight, feet about 12 inches apart, trunk erect with palms beside buttocks. Touch chin to chest, then lean head backwards as far as possible, breathe in deeply as you raise your body so your knees bend, arms remain straight, trunk horizontal, arms and lower legs perpendicular to floor. Tense all your muscles, then relax and breathe out fully as you return to original position; continue this rhythm of deep breathing as you rest between repetitions.

RITE NUMBER FIVE

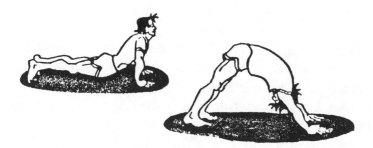

Start face down to floor supported by straight arms perpendicular to the floor. Your hands and feet should be about two feet apart, with arms and legs kept straight throughout. Now lean your head backwards as far as possible, then bend at the hips, breathing in deeply as you raise your body into an inverted V, bringing your chin forward to touch your chest. Tense all your muscles briefly, then breathe out fully as you return to the starting position and again tense all your muscles briefly. Maintain this deep rhythmic breathing between repetitions.

REBIRTHING AND AIDS
by Roger Walther

Rebirthing, also called connected consciousness breathing, is a simple breathing process which can cause profound improvements in your health— not only physical health, but mental, emotional and spiritual health as well. Rebirthing involves breathing in a circular manner while being guided through meditation, visualizations, and other processes by a qualified rebirther who is centered in love, and comes to the experience without negativity about his/her own birth and life. The best way to choose a rebirther is by spending some time with him or her and seeing if you develop trust and love.

A rebirther takes you through approximately ten sessions. During that time, you have the opportunity to breathe and work through a lot of past emotions, feelings, and negative patterns. Spurred by questions and dialogue from your rebirther, you can release birth trauma and painful memories and get in touch with the metaphysical reasons you may have created AIDS in your life. (See Sondra Ray's *Celebration of Breath*, for the appropriate questions concerning rebirthing and healing.) After the ten sessions you will feel comfortable being rebirthed by someone else who has also had ten professional sessions, or by yourself. I recommend after your first ten sessions of one a week that you do the rebirthing process every day for a month, by yourself or with someone else. It is more powerful having someone with you who is non-judgmental and loving toward you and your dis-ease.

On a physical level, rebirthing oxygenates the blood. This is important because many viruses and disease-causing organisms are anaerobic, and will die without carbon dioxide from the blood. It also cleanses, revitalizes, and rejuvenates the cells. This type of breathing is also good to do throughout the day and when hiking, bicycling, jogging, or just walking.

On an emotional level, you have the opportunity to release old anger, fear, resentment, etc. You are able to tap into the inner joy that is your birthright. You will find yourself smiling more and loving yourself and others more.

On a mental level, you release old negative thought patterns like "I'm not good enough," or "I'm not loved or wanted," by seeing where these patterns come from. Rebirthing erases the old mental tapes we run over and over through our minds, and you choose new thoughts by reprogramming your mind with affirmations, meditations, visualizations, and chants.

On a spiritual level, you can get in touch with your higher self and feelings of being one with all that is. Many of us in the gay community have not only rejected organized religion, but also any spirituality, often seeing them as one and the same. By the rebirthing and breathing process, we are able to heal this separation from our spiritual selves, thus discovering our own spirituality and making ourselves whole and complete.

My personal experiences with rebirthing have been profound. My AIDS condition is in remission or healed. (I almost died from pneumocystis in December of 1985.) My blood is normal and my T-cells are healthy. My T-cell count increases daily and my symptoms have disappeared. I have been on a macrobiotic diet, and have taken acupuncture treatments and lymphatic cleanses.

I love my high energy and am enthusiastic about this process called rebirthing. I have been professionally trained to do rebirthing for others.

Rebirthing

"It does have a rather odd name. It isn't a religion or even a therapy. Rebirthing is the art of expanding your sense of well-being and enjoyment. It benefits all of your experience. It is an easy and enjoyable skill you can learn to do for yourself."

—Ann Leonard, *The Five Elements of Rebirthing,* 1986

REBIRTHING RESOURCES

Leonard School of Integrative Rebirthing
2224 - 17th Avenue
San Francisco, CA 94116
(415) 753-0370

Leonard Orr
Consciousness Village
Campbell Hot Springs
P.O. Box 234
Sierraville, CA 96126
(916) 994-8984
(916) 994-3677

Books to read for more information: See Bibliography.

"Brian Mitchell"

I am a gay man in my middle thirties. I am a city person, now living in New York, and previously in Chicago.

There are many advantages to living in a city. One is that you can be anonymous. You need not account to other individuals or groups as you do in small towns. In a city, you can associate with whomever you choose, and avoid others. Of course, it helps if you work for yourself.

I work in the field of graphic arts and advertising, and operate my own business. I communicate only with people of my own choice. Therefore, I am not burdened by a hostile society.

Another advantage to living in the city is that state-of-the-art information on any subject in the world is available. Many types of practitioners are working in a big city.

AIDS is a big subject, and I already knew quite a bit

about AIDS by the time I was diagnosed, without researching it deliberately.

On April 1, 1987, I was diagnosed by Dr. Dan Williams of New York City as having Kaposi's sarcoma. The culprit was two K.S. lesions on the bottoms of my feet.

There is no way to describe the rush of feeling. All the negative information the media was putting out daily to the public rushed into my mind. I bought the fear. I immediately thought of my lover and the possibility that I could have given him the disease. I was shocked, confused, and very frightened. I kept picturing myself covered with lesions like others I have known. I became aware of my mortality.

Dr. Williams arranged a biopsy, and the lesions were removed. The drug Dapsone was prescribed for me, but I had heard that it lowers one's blood count. They wanted me to take it every day, but I didn't take it at all. I didn't want to start putting toxins inside my body.

Because of living in New York City and the people I associate with, I got positive information on alternative, natural treatments very quickly.

My family lives in California, and I let them know what was happening. My mother and my brother Rob came to see me as soon as they could. Rob is a nutritionist and has such total confidence in the healing aspects of diet and herbs that he convinced my mother and me that this disease could be handled, that I did not have to die from it. He relieved me of all or most of my anxiety, giving me a strong feeling of hope which comforted my mother. I began to see a positive path, and I went for it. My zest for life is very strong. I just needed to know that it was possible to deal with this disease. I took another look at what I had to do to stay alive. I had bought the fear once, but would not do that again.

Before the diagnosis, my business life was interesting. I liked to set up graphic arts and advertising businesses. I would start a business, either alone or with a partner, get it going, watch it grow and then go on to the next project. This activity was an outlet for my creative energies. My work allowed me to meet interesting people and to find new challenges.

But in my personal life, I was like a leaf in the wind—scattered. I was sometimes promiscuous. My eating habits were variable. Sometimes I would like myself enough to eat well. At other times it didn't matter what I ate. I had periods of depression and would sometimes find myself unable to function. There was no problem with drugs or alcohol. I have never smoked cigarettes, but I did smoke marijuana.

Over a period of years, I contracted gonorrhea at least four times. Each time the disease was treated with antibiotics. At one time, I had sexually-transmitted hepatitis. I was not given any drugs but was put on total bed rest. I'm not certain I allowed this disease to heal properly before resuming my active life. I'm sure my immune system was weakened.

Once the initial shock of having AIDS had passed, and my brother Rob arrived with his good news, I threw myself into a health-related regimen. I started eating food high in water content like brown rice. I used the herbs Golden Seal and Echinacea with Vitamin C, Vitamin E, multi-vitamins, and acidophilus. I started seeing a health practitioner, Dr. Emanuel Revici, here in New York City. He is a medical doctor and has been treating cancer patients with non-toxic methods, which medical doctors rarely do. AIDS patients have been flocking to him because of his non-toxic treatments. He has had brilliant results with his cancer patients, and people with AIDS are hopeful that this same success will happen for them. I entered an experimental program with this doctor where for two weeks I got injections of a substance he developed that is composed of dead anti-bodies from AIDS patients. It acts like a homeopathic remedy, and is based on the theory that "like cures like." When I got the injections, I had slight symptoms for a short while, and then I felt just great. I began the injections at the same time I made the drastic changes in my diet, so I'm not certain which was more responsible for my T-cell count going up to 540. It certainly made me feel fine when that happened.

That type of injection was stopped, and I took lipids instead. They made me feel wonderful.

I learned that with K.S., one's blood counts may go up and down like a roller coaster, and so I was not to be concerned if that happened.

There was more to my visits at Dr. Revici's office than just physical treatment. On the day of my treatments, I usually arrived at his office early in the morning. I spent hours there talking with other PWA's who were there to see Dr. Revici. We discussed whatever medication was being given since each patient is different, and also various aspects of healing. They were a positive group of people, and I needed psychological support.

My friends behaved predictably. Those who cry easily did. Then we banded together and took a positive approach. It was fortunate that I received much positive information concerning my disease so soon after my diagnosis. A friend came to see me at least once a week to make sure I had plenty of healthful food and that I wanted to eat it. I didn't have a hospital stay to pay for, and didn't take traditional medication, so the cost to me was minimal. My insurance took care of most of it. Good friends helped me financially.

I became connected with Tony Smith and "The Great Pretenders." It was a very positive experience and continues to be. I have made new and meaningful friendships among the PWA's whom I have met. I sense a strong support around me.

I don't know if AIDS is sexually transmitted or not, really. I'm kind of torn about that. My approach to my own illness is to assume that AIDS is sexually transmitted. I have been in a relationship for some time now. My lover is HIV positive. The disease has changed our lives in that we are very careful of bodily fluids. I realize that a person can be re-infected through sexual contact, and that fact is always in the back of my mind. I don't think the physical aspect of AIDS is all there is to it. I believe some people have a will to live and some people don't care much about life. It's not caring that causes their deaths.

I've been talking to PWAs, counseling them on nutrition, and talking to them about their mental attitudes and their will to live. You can see that it just doesn't exist for some people. But there are moments when you can look into a person's eyes and see there a strong will to live. You know that that person can survive this illness.

Most people are doing the traditional medical course of treatment. They are taking immuno-suppressive drugs and are breaking down. They are getting one symptom taken care of but opening themselves up to many more.

To me, the most important aspect of healing is a solid commitment to living. I think that works if a patient isn't too sick. Even then, I'm convinced there are many people who get themselves off the treatment drugs and start dealing with the disease in a more realistic way. One cannot successfully treat immuno-suppressive diseases with immuno-suppressive drugs.

I realize I have not mentioned a religious life. I can only say there is nothing there for me. Not before this disease, nor since. So, I just won't say any more about that.

Another thing I have become aware of is my involvement with the present. This disease has added a new dimension to my life and the things I am learning, because solving its challenge fascinates me. My quest for health is taking me down paths I had not considered before. But there is always fear in the back of my mind, and I must live with it. I found that the only way I could do battle with this virus was to change my lifestyle completely. And I did.

I believe I have become much healthier because of the changes AIDS has made in my life.

Although I cannot see all the ways I have changed, I

know I have changed. I am a different person.

I have rather vague plans for the future; the present is so immediate. The constant thought of my mortality sits right beside the thought of how to get totally healthy. I am very concerned with getting information to others who suffer. A very serious consideration in my mind these days is how to make a long term commitment—to work and to a relationship. I think a lifestyle based on commitment is very positive.

There is also the thought of getting out of New York, to a house somewhere and perhaps a different life altogether, but that has not had time to manifest as yet.

WHAT "BRIAN MITCHELL" DID

• He was open-minded to new ideas. He did not let inappropriate and erroneous information confound his thinking.

• He listened to a nutritionist who convinced him that proper nutrition with wholesome foods and diet supplementation would change his blood chemistry and give his body energy to heal itself.

• He allowed time enough for his healing, realizing that natural, holistic methods take time.

• He sought out non-toxic treatment. He was open to whatever worked. He refused to allow immuno-suppressive drugs to be administered to him.

• He talked to other individuals who had conquered AIDS, found out what they did, and deductively and rationally created his own therapies.

• He did not believe all that he read and heard from the media.

• He shared his experience with others, uniting and making a strong bond with a group of individuals who also wanted healing. He learned to help others.

• "Brian Mitchell" decided that he was going to get well, and he did.

Note: "Brian Mitchell" is connected with "The Great Pretenders."

THE GREAT PRETENDERS, INC. of New York is a men's team committed to bring love, success, and happiness to all men through teamwork.

Headquartered at 149 West 12th Street in New York City, the team is composed of a core of five founding members and includes other men on both ad hoc and continuing bases. The team was born out of the "Men, Sex, and Power" weekend in early 1984. Since that time, it has developed the trust and powerful, committed intimacy that appears to be so rare among men today, and for which there is great hunger and a tremendous opportunity.

As an organization dedicated to bringing the full power and freedom of men to be a positive, life-giving, life-sustaining force on the planet today, The Great Pretenders focus their work and projects in four main areas: the media, community projects, healing, and training and consultation.

They believe that real healing comes from the mind, and involves reprogramming one's thinking. Their first premise is the denial of doubt, fear, and hopelessness. They taught "Brian Mitchell" that undoubtedly AIDS is partly a fear-induced disease, and that fear obsession can cause biological, physical, and psychological changes in the body. Reprogramming their thinking and expression of feelings and confronting their emotional states is a catharsis, purifying both mind and body, because when one lets go of the fear, oftentimes the disease goes with it.

ALL'S WELL is an organization whose members are committed to the transformation of our ability to create well being. We assert the following: that Good Health can be created by every individual depending on the conversation he or she has with the self. Having a negative conversation with the subconscious mind regarding health and healing can actually allow illness to develop. We also assert that showing people how to shift their conversation to a healing mode can reduce the incidence of illness in the world.

While our focus is on the condition called AIDS, *any illness* can be transformed. In general, people who have AIDS or ARC hold a set of beliefs that foster physical self-abuse. Such abuse may take various forms, such as use and abuse of drugs, having poor nutritional and dietary habits, engaging in unsafe sexual practices or getting inadequate rest. Physical self-abuse is combined with "death threats"—that is, the belief that once contracted, the HIV virus will eventually destroy the immune system. This belief is promoted by the medical community, the media and the political establishment, all of whom hold control over knowledge of and development of a cure for this disease.

Putting total faith in these power structures leads to the individual holding an intrinsic belief that he or she is powerless to fight the progression from HIV-positive to full-blown AIDS.

The medical experts would have us totally rely on drugs, chemotherapy and other invasive techniques to alter the body. These therapies actually do damage to an already weakened immune system.

So, AIDS = self abuse + death threats + immuno-suppressive therapy.

"All's Well" has been created to shift our culture's perspective from one of the individual as victim to that of personal responsibility for Good Health. Our commitment to improving people's physical, emotional and spiritual well being can help support others to not only stay alive, but also to make informed choices about their health. There are people who have used an HIV-positive test result or an AIDS/ARC diagnosis to dramatically improve their health, despite such test results and diagnoses. The power to heal, to cure, is within each person's grasp.

ALL'S WELL
40 West 38 Street
Fourth Floor
New York, NY 10018
(212) 382-0771

"Steven Greer"

In the past six years, since my diagnosis of AIDS, my life has made a complete turnaround. I am 32 now, healthy and full of enthusiasm about my present life and my future. There are no drugs in my life now.

I believe that AIDS is caused by a combination of drugs and different viruses that come in contact with those chemicals. Combined, they affect the immune system drastically. I believe that AIDS is a lifestyle disease, and is sexually transmitted. Being sexually promiscuous has something to do with acquiring AIDS.

I believe that I got AIDS because I wasn't living right. I was using various kinds of drugs, kept late hours, and was very hard on my body. I was a heavy cocaine user, and smoked marijuana and used amylnitrates occasionally, but no IV drugs.

Once I had a light case of hepatitis which weakened my liver. I was sick for three or four months. I did not take antibiotics, but simply used rest to recover.

In 1981, I was diagnosed as having Burkitt's lymphoma. This is a form of cancer which is considered fatal. I had chemotherapy for it; the doctors gave me from three to six months to live. Instead, I used the protocol at St. Jude's International Clinic in Mexico, and the result was—I was free of the disease.

In February, 1983, I was diagnosed as having Kaposi's sarcoma on my upper palate, and AIDS. They did a biopsy on the KS. They suspected that I had had AIDS all that time. They had called it Burkitt's disease because they did not know much about AIDS at that time.

In all of 1984 and 1985, I appeared to be clear of disease. But in August of 1986, I was diagnosed again as having KS on the left calf. They gave me Interferon. This caused fever, chills, fatigue, headaches. They did exploratory surgery on me in Los Angeles. The disease was now located in my lower intestine, the abdominal area. They removed the tumor and took out a foot of the lower intestine and started me on chemotherapy. The only drug given me was Interferon. It is very expensive, but as it was experimental, I did not pay for it. This was a special research program.

When I first learned that I had AIDS, I went into a depression. Being very sick—with the threat of early death at 31—really made me stop and think. I decided to totally change my lifestyle, and GOT WELL!

X-rays now show nothing wrong inside. In August, 1987, I had a CAT scan, which was an X-ray of my entire body—a highly technological process—and it showed that everything is fine. I also had tests for my T-cell count.

The doctors were surprised at my recovery. Every time I would go to one of them, he would look at me as if I were a ghost. He would ask: "How ARE you?"—amazed at how well I was doing. My recovery is due in part to the therapy at St.

Jude's, but largely to my complete change of lifestyle and way of thinking.

Now I count my blessings. I consider everything I have and how lucky I am—not only because I am still alive, but because I have the outlook that life is worth living.

There was something I needed to learn—how to be a better person; how to become more aware of my body and what it needs. I have started to take control of my life.

How can people protect themselves from getting AIDS? By having "safe sex" or self-sex. Is "safe sex" really safe? It is, 95% of the time. But there is always that 5% margin, and I would not do it.

In my experience with AIDS, I have lost many friends. The disease showed me who my friends really are.

To what do I owe my recovery? I am a Christian; I believe in God. My lifestyle has changed dramatically. I have stopped all drugs, even stopped the social drinking. I do not do the things I used to do. My sex life has changed; I do not do anal intercourse now. In fact, my sex life is with myself (masturbation)—nothing else. My thinking about myself has changed, absolutely. I have a more positive outlook on life. I am a better person now, because of what has happened to me. I feel I now have control over my body, and have overcome the disease. My mental ability and calmness are much greater than they used to be.

My family had a great deal to do with my recovery. They are religious. I have a big family, and I love it—the closeness with a large family, in this small town. I live four houses from my mother; my brother lives across the street from her. So with the family in three nearby houses, we are close in space, but also close in our hearts.

The love that friends gave me helped. Also, I have done a great deal of Transcendental Meditation, and finally, your book, Bianca and Scott—*CONQUERING AIDS NOW!* I had heard about alternative therapies, but did not quite understand them until I read your book.

While I was in the healing process, what seemed to make the disease worse was being alone. This caused a depression. Fear plays a big part in this—the fear of death.

You can't expect doctors to heal you with drugs. You must take control of your mind and your body. Your mind can tell your body what it wants to manifest! I was fortunate in having all those factors—all those pluses in my life—an early background of prayer, church, and a loving family—all of which I could return to. Not every Person With AIDS has all that, or is so fortunate. And yet the potential is always there for him—if he will reach out and take it. Friends and help will come—if one reaches out.

My life has changed in so many ways, since I got AIDS. It started changing when I became determined to live.

I am a vegetarian now. I decided to purify my diet after reading a book a friend sent me—*Living with Cancer*. This was in 1983. I am taking supplements now—Vitamins A, B, C, zinc, and magnesium.

As to working, I was a bartender in Los Angeles before I got sick. Now I am not working for a living, although I am able to. I have a small garden and a huge yard, with flower beds. Living in a small town helps me a lot. There is less stress than in cities. There is cleaner air, and you can see the stars at night. I returned to the town where I grew up. I have found my old friends from my youth.

I do want to go back to work. There is a family business, in trucking oil. My brother is in it; our father left it to us.

Another positive force in my recovery was my doctor, a woman named Mateel Graham, at Parkland Hospital in Dallas. She helped relieve my fear of death. She never told me: "You're going to die," but "We're going to make it!"

I took control of my thinking, with this doctor's help. I hear that some Persons With Aids have suicidal thoughts. I did not. I was always positive and confident that I would recover and live. Of course, I had my ups and downs. The drugs caused fatigue, a high fever, some nausea, and occasionally diarrhea. But because of wonderful Dr. Graham, who helped change my thinking, I felt well about four months after I was diagnosed in 1983. I wish that all doctors had the same confidence and compassion of Dr. Graham. She is an ideal doctor.

My decision was to get well. I knew I would make it. It was a conviction I had inside of me.

I found that one must give attention to both a spiritual life and the physical body. My spiritual life is important. I attend church, sing in the choir, and say prayers. I have said many a prayer in my crisis and in all of my life.

I was from this small town. Then I went to the big city, and got into all kinds of trouble with a destructive lifestyle. Now I am back in my small town, with a purified life. I guess you could compare me with "The Prodigal Son" in the New Testament parable.

I suppose I left my home town for the big cities to conceal my homosexuality from my family, and to experience total freedom. I found out that total freedom can be destructive to life.

There is a great deal about AIDS in the magazines, newspapers, and on television. I believe they are not telling us enough: not advising us how to take care of our bodies, not teaching prevention. We must give our bodies the nutrients they need, and not overstress them. Then there is positive thinking—the mental and the spiritual aspects of man. Who is teaching this? Not the schools, not the media. The churches are teaching about the mind and the spirit. It is all in books—for those who seek and find them. But many persons do not seek, and do not read, and do not find.

While I was in Houston, I was referred to a Dr. Anderson, and went to several group therapy sessions while there. A number of AIDS patients were in the same room, and it seemed they were telling me their problems. I didn't like it. I had my own problems; I didn't need to hear theirs. It is not a good form of therapy, in my opinion. I was depressed after each session, so I did not attend further.

Some Persons With AIDS are saying, "I don't give a damn. I don't care whether I live or die." Some people are strong and some are weak. Some have a great love for life, and some do not.

It is being said that God is punishing gays for what they are doing. I do not feel that is true.

My family did not know that I was gay until I got AIDS. That put pressure on me to explain my homosexuality. My sister said to me, " I don't understand it." I replied, "I don't either, but that is the way I am."

It all started when I was a child. I was sick a lot, with asthma and other ailments. I suffered much as a child. I was abused sexually and mentally, when I was eight years old. The man was a next-door neighbor. He was nice and I trusted him. I knew that what he was doing to me was wrong, but I never told my parents. I have learned that this is very common. Children are afraid to speak out about sexual abuse. They feel confused and guilty.

Some people don't know how to show love. My parents were alcoholic and did not, could not, show me the affection I needed. While in high school, I had sex with a man of my own choosing. I knew it was wrong, but I liked it. He gave me the love and affection I was starved for. My later life was affected a great deal by this. It caused me to become a homosexual.

But now, as I said, I am not having any sex. I've had to concentrate on recovery.

People who don't make it—what are they doing wrong? They are not caring about themselves or others sufficiently. They are not taking responsibility for their sickness. They are not having enough hope. I would advise them, in three words: "Keep the faith!"

WHAT "STEVEN GREER" DID

• He wanted to live. He made a decision to get well, and knew he would recover.

• He sought out an alternative metabolic therapy in Mexico, and this was a primary factor in his healing.

• He had confidence in his doctor, and she had compassion for him. She relieved him of the fear of death.

• He took control of his thinking, his body, and his life.

• He realized that one cannot separate the spiritual life from the body—that life is one.

• He learned to give his body the proper nutrients and not overstress it.

• He became a vegetarian, when he found the vegetarian diet to be a purer, more healthful diet.

• He decided to purify his body, after reading *Conquering AIDS Now!* He did much reading, on health and spiritual subjects.

• He started taking supplements, and learned which ones were best for him.

• He developed a small garden; he grows fruits and vegetables.

• He cultivated reverence for his body. He learned how to become more aware of his body and what it needs.

• He stopped all drugs, even social drinking, and all destructive habits.

• He has a more positive, happy outlook on life.

• He is a better person now, because of what happened to him.

• His family supported him in every way, and wanted him to recover.

• He returned to the town of his childhood. He found there less stress than in cities, cleaner air, and fewer temptations.

• He found his old friends from youth, and made new friendships in his church.

• He had something to look forward to, a family business to develop.

• He learned to be calm and mentally stable.

• "Steven Greer" learned positive thinking, discovered spiritual truths, and had a spiritual rebirth.

ST. JUDE'S INTERNATIONAL CLINIC

Jimmy Keller, Director, advised the authors that in addition to "Steven Greer," a Los Angeles chiropractor who took the therapies at St. Jude's also recovered from AIDS.

The clinic states that it "offers a remarkably successful metabolic treatment program for cancer and other degenerative diseases."

Address: 911 Television, Tijuana, C.C., Mexico
Telephone: (706) 681-3026

"John Davies"

When I was eight years old my family sent me away to a boarding school, and I spent the next seven years there. I don't know why my parents sent me away, but they did. I have a brother and sister, but I have never lived with them. We love each other, but when we meet it takes a long time for me to get close to them.

I became sexually active at about nine years of age. I practiced group masturbation with the boys. There was no serious sex. No penetration, no hugs or kisses and no one to hold. It was a kind of little-boy lust. At that time, I established myself as a homosexual. I found the feeling very satisfying partly because I think it was the only feeling I had. At least, it was the strongest feeling. My early sexual indulgences and intensity of my feelings caused me to become confused. There was no one I could talk to about it. At the time, I didn't even know there should be someone to talk to. My confusion gave birth to a negative thinking pattern that was to follow me through my life.

When I left boarding school, I went to live with my father. Living with my dad was difficult. I did not feel that he really liked me. It could have been my own lack of love for myself that fit in well with my negative thinking patterns established so early. My father died not long ago, and the problems that existed between us were never resolved.

As a teen-ager in high school, I felt very disconnected from the world. I had no ambition to study. There was no motivation to try to accomplish anything. That's when I found the party concept, and I took up partying with a vengeance. I smoked pot every day for a couple of years, and I drank anything I could get my hands on. I dropped acid at least twelve times in two years, but the time came when I realized that I would have to do something to clean up my life, so I joined the Air Force.

I stayed in the Air Force for four years. I spent two years in the Netherlands and two years in Colorado. I was given a battery of vaccines and antibiotics. The vaccines were given to me to help me, not to hurt me, but I believe they caused my immune system to become suppressed.

While I was in the Air Force, I felt I had a healthy life. I ate balanced meals, meat-and-potato style, but I didn't know of any other way of eating. I did a lot of biking, and I took saunas and felt pretty good about my health. I was quite thin, but I felt good. About this time, I was seeing a girl, but without telling anyone, I would sneak away to the baths to indulge myself sexually. Actually, it was at this time that I realized I was a bi-sexual.

At this point, the Air Force sent me to the Netherlands. Amsterdam is a beautiful city, but very decadent. I discovered a very active gay population in the Netherlands. Sex is a product on the market place. Everything seems to be out in the open, and no one seems bothered much about it. At least, there aren't people who judge and point fingers at others. I was very comfortable in the Netherlands. I had a certain drive for decadence, at least a willingness to involve myself. The European lifestyle accommodated my desires. Perhaps sex has a market value in every city, and only the buyers and sellers know the price.

During my stay in the Air Force, I became a photographer. I was "paid military," so life was not unpleasant for me while I was abroad. I still felt healthy and was living out my fantasies of decadence. After two years in the Netherlands, I returned to the States.

I was sent to Colorado. I joined a ski team, and worked hard at photography. I didn't have a high rank, so there was only so much I could do as a photographer. But I was beginning to be given work that was perhaps a little too important for a person of my level. I don't know whether this was the cause of my problem with the people I worked with or not, but I had a terrible time getting along with them. I was really glad when my time was up, and I could get out of the service and carry on with my life.

I was eager to be on my own. It would be the first time in my life that I had ever been independent. I planned to go to Los Angeles to try to get into the motion picture studios as a photographer and to continue my photographic studies. I hoped to gradually work my way to the position of Director of Photography and make films. I still want to work in photography. I am taking courses in photography at a local community college. My studies were important to me before AIDS, and they are important now. That's one thing that hasn't changed.

I was totally unprepared for life in the big city. I had very little money, and I knew hardly anyone. I enrolled as a full-time student. I took whatever jobs I could find to keep going. I paid no attention to my health, seldom eating properly. I did not recognize the need for nourishing food to sustain good health. I had the idea that if I could get through this difficult period, I could find a way to fulfill my dream of creative photography. I think I have the "photographer's eye" or visual response that makes for a photographic artist. Photography is an exciting art, and I believe that I can develop into becoming one of its artists.

Unfortunately, the fast life in the city seduced me quickly. I started working in night clubs until late. I also started experimenting with drugs. I became sexually very active. For almost eight months, I would do cocaine at least three times a week. Cocaine is a very expensive habit. I worked harder and longer hours to support my lifestyle. When I ate, I didn't pay any attention to what I was eating. I began to let everything go; my life took a negative turn. I became weaker and began to feel tired all the time. I just had no energy at all, but continued to force myself to do things that I felt had to be done. I continued to avoid the real issues by indulging in sex and drugs. I allowed my health to deteriorate, and did nothing to stop it. I could see what was happening to me, but I didn't know what to do. AIDS was unfamiliar to me until sometime in 1985. At that time, a man I knew and had worked with, who lived in my apartment building, was very sick. He died of pneumocystis. I heard this news but didn't know anything about the disease. I didn't know I was in the high risk group. I thought I was fine.

It was about this time that I began to feel really bad. At first, I put it off as unimportant, believing that I was just working too hard and doing too much, but the fatigue became worse. I often became quite sick. There was no way of ignoring it any longer, so I went to see Dr. Gorlitsky, an internist in Santa Monica. He did the ELISA and the Western Blot tests and the results showed AIDS positive. He also did a CBC, and he told me not to worry, as my white blood count was good. I know that some doctors will hospitalize you for a positive AIDS diagnosis.

I think the reason Dr. Gorlitsky didn't hospitalize me at

that time was that my white blood count was good, and I was not showing any symptoms. At least, that is what he said. He told me to eat properly, live a healthy life, and I would be all right. As for me, I felt just horrible. I thought a doctor would give me more information than that, but I think Dr. Gorlitsky did the best he could. You must recognize the limitations of medical doctors where alternative treatments are concerned. Part of the medical-drug complex, they refuse to consider that anyone or anything can heal other than traditional-medicine doctors and their prescription drugs. The people of this country are very trusting of the big authority figures. We want them to tell us what is good for us. Besides, we want a pill to cure all our ills—and quickly—so we cooperate with the orthodox doctors to keep them and ourselves in ignorance.

The effort that it takes to break through that ignorance is profound. I feel that those who survive this disease will be people with a very powerful will to live and function normally—and a willingness to learn the methods available for achieving these goals. I am one of those people; I believed I could be healed. And so it proved.

I was diagnosed on December 1, 1986 as having AIDS. I was stunned. Confusion as to how to "eat right," and "lead a healthy life" almost overcame me. I knew changes had to be made and fast, but I didn't know what to do. I felt so sick. I had hard nodes in my throat. I tried to call all the hotlines I could find to see what I could learn. They told me to eat right, maintain a meditative state as much as possible, and most important, to avoid stress.

I had never had any religious belief up to this time, so there was no spiritual comfort available to me. My brother, sister, and I were not close, so I could not turn to them. My father had died. My mother came through for me as she always has. We are very close, and she has helped me a great deal through this.

In February of 1987, I developed a terrible cold and went

to the UCLA Clinic. I saw a Dr. Wolf. He looked me over and said there was nothing wrong with me. He is an AIDS specialist. When I confronted him with the AIDS positive diagnosis, he said that I displayed no symptoms; therefore, there was no treatment he could give me to relieve my distress. Dr. Wolf arranged for some blood work to be done. When the tests came back, the nurse told me the prognosis wasn't good. She said I was on the borderline. My condition could develop into K.S. or pneumocystis and full-blown AIDS. My T-cell count was 357. The blood test showed a T-4 at 357 with a T-8 cell count of 799 with an inverted T-ratio of .45. I asked the nurse what I should do. She told me to "keep healthy." They were not much help. They could give me all the numbers, and that was fine, but now it was up to me to find a way to heal myself. I see in retrospect that I was being protected, perhaps by a divine power, as the medics did not urge me to take or even offered drug treatments.

I was feeling really terrible. I had no energy, and I was terribly depressed. One night as I was lying in bed listening to the radio, I happened to tune into a program with a psychic called Mina Khalil. I decided to call her. She gave me a consultation and didn't even charge me. She also sent me a tape that was very, very informative. She was the one who told me that I should take the route of natural healing. "You will be healed," she said. "Carry this message to others who still suffer. If you do this, you will become notable."

She gave me the direction I needed. I think I had been moving in the direction of natural therapies, and perhaps her counsel to take this path was what I needed to hear. She told me something that I already knew within myself. I guess that is what psychics do, and why people go to them. I know I am very grateful for her consultation, the tape she sent me, and for her caring and compassionate attitude.

At some point, I wandered into the One Life health food store in Santa Monica. They sell health foods, books, herbs and many things of interest to a person like me. I started poking around the herbs because I seemed to be drawn to their healing capabilities. The psychic set great store by Golden Seal, and I started to learn more about herbs as I embarked upon this great adventure of healing.

I found the book *Love, Medicine and Miracles* by Bernie Siegel, M.D. He writes about the positive mental attitude of cancer patients. He discusses the will to live and explains visualization techniques. He believes as I do that the will to live is the most important factor in a cure.

Next, I discovered your book. (*Conquering AIDS Now!* by Scott Gregory and Bianca Leonardo.) I bought the book and read it through that same day. Many new doors opened! My life has completely changed since that day. I reversed the downward trend into illness.

I studied diet on all levels and developed my own nutritional program. I do not eat anything with chemicals in it. I do not eat food which has been preserved or processed in any way. I have discovered that dairy foods are poison to me, so I don't partake of them. I still eat some chicken and fish, but compared to the amount of fresh vegetables and fruit, the amount of flesh I eat is negligible. I bake my own bran muffins and my own bread. I shop at very special stores and search out the best products. I press my own fresh vegetable and fruit juices. My new diet initiated the detoxification period that is necessary for a healing to happen.

I began to study other natural therapies and found acupuncture an excellent method for relieving pain and distress. I learned about massage, herbs, rebirthing, meditation, and nutrition. I re-discovered a spiritual life; I returned to the church. I am a Catholic, and although I know that people with AIDS are looked down upon by the church, I feel that the Divine is concerned with us and our healing ourselves. So I go to church.

I experienced an infinite awareness. My mind, experiences, and emotions opened up. In some way, I began to tap into energies that were previously dormant. I cannot deny these unknown factors exist, because I have experienced them.

I began to understand that there are no established procedures or drugs to deal with this illness. The medical establishment is baffled. The orthodox medical profession uses drugs like AZT as a placebo to calm desperate people and make it look as though the "establishment" is doing something. AZT is a terrible drug. I wouldn't touch it with a ten-foot pole. If I were to break my leg, I would go to a medical doctor to have it set, but would not go for this illness. Even if I could afford it, I wouldn't use medical treatments for AIDS.

In the field of natural healing, I find many practitioners who are willing to treat me whether I can pay or not. I find the herbs incredibly inexpensive, and they work. I have a deep compassion for people working in the field of natural healing. They do it for their love of mankind—not for profit.

The American Medical Association is a very powerful organization and is married to the pharmaceutical companies. Thus the power is increased. I recently heard that the average cost for an AIDS patient for hospitalization and drugs is $50,000 per year. That does not include care, just hospitalization and drugs. That being the case, there is no way we can deny that AIDS involves big money. History shows us that there are many people willing and eager to make money from other people's suffering. The AIDS situation with its suffering and stress has proved that many people of this caliber still exist.

Imagine what it would be like if the American Medical Association joined with all the healing practitioners on the natural path. Knowledge would be shared. How much simpler it would be to find the healing modalities needed for different illnesses.

Being sick is not fun. I'm on my own here in Los Angeles and it's been tough, very tough. I do my best not to get into a state of stress, but it is difficult. I am grateful for the help I have received from so many sources. I am aware that each of us is different. I realize that there are many, many variables, but I think that each of us needs to clean the toxins out of his body. How you choose to perform this cleansing is, of course, up to you. When your body is thoroughly cleansed (and this can take a long time), then it is time to rebuild the tissues that have been depleted. To rebuild your tissues, choose the method best suited to you. Just remember, you will feel worse before you feel better. Do not become frightened when you find yourself feeling worse. It is part of the cleansing. Of course, don't pay so much attention to the body that you forget the emotions and the mind. The very first step is to recognize how much you want to live.

Recently, I bought a colonic board. I knew I was very toxic. I could feel it, and my illness was evidence of a deep toxicity. Even so, I did not know how toxic I was. This was my first colonic. It left toxins stirred up in my body. I excreted mucus and waste for three days. I felt just terrible. It is necessary to rest after a colonic, especially the first one, and I did rest. I felt really sick. But there is a difference in this kind of "feeling sick," because I know it is the prelude to feeling better. Recognizing how toxic my system really was motivated me to do everything I could to cleanse my system. Seeing how toxic I was frightened and amazed me. No wonder I got sick.

I think Oriental medicine has much to offer, with its ancient methods of healing. I find I respond well to acupuncture and, of course, my beloved herbs. But, I will definitely use the colonic again during another period of detoxification. I think this is the order of healing: a cleansing colonic, good nutrition, herbs, and acupuncture. This is good for me, but nothing is permanent. I am open to adjustments in the regimen.

To completely detoxify may take a while, but I am persistent. I know I will succeed, and find a level of health I have not known before. I thought I was healthy when I was in the Air Force, but now I know that there is another level of good health, the true level. I am reaching for it.

As to my personal life, I have decided to live a nonsexual life. I believe the virus is sexually transmitted, and, considering that I fell victim to AIDS, I decided I didn't want to endanger anyone else. I don't believe there is any such thing as "safe" sex for anyone at this time in history. We are all at risk. Heterosexuals as well as homosexuals are subject to this disease. Some groups may be in a higher risk category than others, but we are all vulnerable. I don't want to spread this illness. I don't know what my future attitude toward sex will be since I know that re-infection is possible. As far as I'm concerned, to act out sex would be to indulge myself or fool myself, or both. I have learned to respect my body.

I have become a totally different person since I was diagnosed. I now realize that we are not invincible. Our lives are fragile.

I have become aware of spiritual forces and energies unknown to me before. I am much more open to new things: approaches, great persons with a message. This is a big world; I'm just one person, but I can make a difference by helping others to solve their problems as I have been helped in solving my own.

I am closer to my family than I have ever been or thought I would ever be. I find I care a great deal about other people, and I am sensitive to them. I spend lots of time on the phone with PWA's, and I have met and learned from a number of people in the field of natural healing. I have changed in so many ways, it's impossible to count them.

You must be very honest with yourself, have a positive attitude, and determine how far you are willing to go in changing your life to defeat this illness.

My work at school is still very important to me. I have visions of creating a healing environment of some kind. The whole dream has not taken form as yet. As I learn more, I will have more of a message to carry to those who still suffer. I know I must yet investigate the benefits and methods of exercise for myself. Somehow, I would like to incorporate photography with a healing environment. I don't know how as yet, but I have just begun the journey.

The most important thing I can say to a PWA is that there is hope. Don't believe the negative publicity. There are many things you can do to make yourself more comfortable and eventually bring about a healing.

I want to thank everyone who has helped me through this period of my life. I feel that I am on the right path for me. I sincerely hope some of the things that I have said will help many in their recovery from this dreaded disease. The truth is that those who are fighting AIDS are not alone, and can recover!

I have done so, and this is my story.

WHAT "JOHN DAVIES" DID

• He realized no "magic bullet" existed to cure him and that taking drugs would not result in a healing.

• He did not listen to the medical generalities on AIDS, or the negative prognoses—"AIDS is invariably fatal."

• He rejected the medical path—drugs, chemotherapy, etc.—all the medical complex has to offer Persons With AIDS—and sought out other avenues for his healing.

• He believed that he could heal himself.

• He knew that self-healing involves good nutrition, leading a healthy lifestyle, and positive thinking.

• He discovered what was going on inside his body.

• He received clear directions of what he needed to do to heal himself.

• He avoided stress.

• He refused to allow the fear of death to develop within himself.

• He listened to audio tapes on natural healing, and was given directions in this path.

• He began to use creative visualization techniques.

• He studied various healthful diets and developed his own nutritional program, including herbs.

• He did not use chemicalized foods or allergy-producing foods.

• He cooked for himself, believing that his kitchen was his own pharmacy. ("Food is the best medicine," counseled Hippocrates, the Father of Medicine, two thousand years ago.)

• He learned about acupuncture, massage, colonics, pain and stress reduction, etc.

• He sought out a spiritual path and developed a spiritual life.

• He discovered the book *Conquering AIDS Now!* (Gregory and Leonardo), and followed its precepts. This healing protocol, both through the book and via personal consultations with Dr. Gregory, resulted in a detoxification of the body, destruction of the virus, and the strengthening of his immune system. He had a complete healing.

• He realized that helping others is very important for a healthy, happy life—and after his healing, he shared himself.

• "John Davies" decided to LIVE, and achieved his goal.

"Bertie Chapin"

In January of 1986 I was hospitalized with pneumocystis pneumonia that confirmed my diagnosis of AIDS. The attending physician in the hospital, the Beekman Downtown Infirmary in New York, was Dr. Schulman. I remained in the hospital about four weeks.

The diagnosis caused some discord in my family. My mother and father are divorced. My father lives in Indiana, and my brother, who is younger than I, lives in Ohio. I have never been close to them. This indifferent relationship still exists despite the fact of my illness.

My homosexuality caused some controversy with aunts, uncles, and a grandmother. The major problem was with my cousins. My family knew, and I assumed my cousins also knew that I was gay, but they did not know. When they found out about my illness, I was banned from their home.

I was prepared for this sort of thing to happen when I revealed that I was gay. The situation just happened eight years late. My father was typically American. He did not like the fact that I was not what I was" supposed to be." When I was a child, I liked playing with dolls, dressing up in feminine clothes, jumping rope and doing things not of a masculine nature. I simply was totally unlike my brother.

I was not unathletic, however. Had I been brought up in a different community, I might have developed gymnastically, because I loved doing cartwheels and hand flips, but the community had no gym for this. I was also an excellent swimmer, and enjoyed it.

My peers in the second grade didn't understand my leanings. I was very good at jumping rope when children were twirling them. I could enter between the ropes and jump all day, loving it, but the boys of my class weren't interested in competing with me.

There was a certain secrecy in my upbringing. I wasn't supposed to display my inclinations. My father disapproved, but my mother understood that my love for playing dress-up was partly because I liked textures of fabrics. She felt that I was creative and enjoyed working with materials, draping them and creating fashion designs. She was correct in her understanding, because I developed into an excellent fashion designer. I consider my childhood as holding the roots not only of my talent and creativity, but of my homosexuality.

During my early years while growing up, I received the usual vaccines given to children for smallpox and measles. I even had an oral polio vaccine. About two months prior to my AIDS diagnosis, I was treated for an amoebic infection and given medication. I don't know what type of parasite I had, or what medication I was given.

It is believed that AIDS is sexually transmitted but, unlike other venereal diseases, it seems as if everything has to be just "right" for it to take hold. I had been denying myself throughout my whole upbringing and I was in a very low emotional state. I was undergoing a very difficult time with my current lover because of a problem of communication. Just prior to this, I had a similar upset with my former lover, resulting in our breaking up. I constantly felt as if no one understood me. Friends seemed to feel that if I understood their point of view, I should negate my own. I had an inner turmoil at the time I received my diagnosis.

I had an on-going flu. I had chronic fatigue. Then I began to show signs of shortness of breath.

In our office, we have two connected floors. I had once been able to run up and down between them. Now the problem was I got out of breath. Finally I couldn't do it at all, and said, "I have to give myself some rest."

I stayed home from work for about a week, but my condition got worse. I grew weaker until I couldn't get up to go to the bathroom. I couldn't get up to prepare food during the day and was only eating when my roommate came home at night and fixed dinner. Consequently, I was losing weight. That is basically the history of my symptoms.

When I was diagnosed, I was scared to find myself in a high risk category, and yet I didn't believe that I filled the "requirements" of being a PWA.

In 1977, I had moved from Cincinnati, Ohio to New York. A few years after moving, friends and I were talking about how promiscuous we had been, trying to remember how many men we might have had sex with. I was literally able to name them all. At that time, there were only about thirty, and since then, I would say I've added perhaps twenty more. I had a two-and-a-half year monogamous relationship with one man. After we broke up, I had another monogamous relationship that lasted another two years or so. So, I would not say that I was really promiscuous. Someone else might say so, but for the gay lifestyle, I certainly was not.

One wonderful summer, I worked on Mackinac Island.

Since it was a resort, everybody was into the swing. One night stands out especially in my memories. It was my first sexual experience. I had really been romanticizing it. I had wanted more than just a one night stand. But it didn't turn out that way. So I decided that if this was the gay life, I didn't want to be gay.

I had no interest in girls at the time—that just didn't happen to me. Then I returned to college and joined a fraternity. I dated a girl, but we never had sex. I continued one-night flings and tricks with men once every two or three months.

Then I met a wonderful woman who had many gay friends. She introduced me to several male couples who had been together for two to three years. It was then I realized that men could have long-term relationships. My girl friend and I broke up, and I came out of the closet.

If I ran into somebody like a trucker who thought I might be a little bit swishy, I just let his attitude tumble off my shoulders. It was actually his problem, not mine.

I used recreational drugs, but not much. Marijuana at times, some cocaine, but not as often as once in two months. Years ago, friends and I used something called Ecstasy, and also Purple Haze. Another time, I did a half a hit of blotter acid, and I think that's about the history of my drug use. I was never an I.V. drug user.

When I was nineteen, I started smoking cigarettes. I smoked for about eleven years and then quit "cold turkey."

Alcohol was another story. Friends and I would go out to bars at least once during the week, and once or twice on the weekend. I would get drunk, but I was always able to walk home.

My AIDS was probably sexually transmitted. Part of my conditioning for the illness, I believe, was the fact that I had been living only half a life. I had been instilled with a sense of lack of self-worth.

I didn't worry consciously about getting AIDS, not considering myself a prime candidate for it, but the thought lurked in the back of my mind. I believe that most of the gay community have such thoughts. We are always wondering who's going to be next.

I was saddened by my diagnosis, but in another way, it almost made me feel good. A simultaneous thought was: "Now you don't have to worry about getting it any more."

The first time I was in the hospital, I was quite ill. My doctor tried to encourage me not to be worried about the diagnosis. He was concerned primarily with curing the pneumonia and getting me back on my feet, then going on to the next step.

When I entered the hospital, I couldn't walk. In fact, I was already being given oxygen. I was receiving Pentamadine, an antiviral drug for the lungs. In addition, I was given medication intravenously, but I'm not sure what it was. I may also have been receiving Flagyl, which is an antibiotic.

Fortunately, I didn't have any side effects from the treatment—from the medical treatment, that is. I was not treated so well by the staff. I understand that the floor I was on was noted for poor treatment. It was really awful. I wasn't officially isolated, but there was a sign posted on the door saying that everybody who came into my room had to wear gloves, mask, and rubber shoes.

The doctors were saying that I might get worse before I got better from the pneumocystis pneumonia, depending on whether they were able to stop it. This wasn't happening. Then suddenly, a couple of days later, I noticed I was having difficulty breathing. One evening, as I was finishing dinner, I fell asleep. My mother and my lover were there with me. They were talking quietly as I dozed off. When I awakened, they noticed that my chest was heaving in labored breathing. Visiting hours were over; it was time for them to leave. We called a nurse and told her what was going on. She looked at my oxygen level, and said, "You just relax, honey." She was a big, black, Haitian woman. This nurse had an attitudinal problem, as did the whole staff on this floor. She repeated, "You're getting exactly what the doctor ordered. Just relax. You'll be fine."

"Look," I remonstrated, "I know that's what the doctor ordered, but something is going wrong. I think something needs to be checked."

She just put her hands on her hips and looked at me and said, "Don't try to tell me what I'm supposed to do." To her my upset was nothing and did not deserve her consideration. Essentially, the nurses believed that no problem could develop between doctor visits.

This overbearing attitude was compensated for by the fact that many of my friends and others put me at the top of their considerations.

A group was being started in New York for PWAs called the Well-Being Group, whose purpose is to awaken our own personal power. They're not as formal as the AIDS Coalition. The members are interested in spiritual awareness and alternatives types of healing.

The group members feel that there is a Power higher than ourselves—an all-inclusive Power. The members tap into this power through meditation, relaxation, and visualization, very much like Louise Hay's teachings. We had a person within the group, Annette Maxbery, who was very good at channeling. She was, and continues to be, wonderfully supportive.

The whole group worked together, each supporting the other. The first section met once a week for ten weeks, the second section for twelve weeks. The program was based upon the kind of work that Carl and Stephanie Simonton, cancer specialists, have done. It was a small, informal group, privately funded.

We delved into and discussed various alternative methods. We talked about nutritious macrobiotic food. We had masseurs and acupuncturists coming to the meetings. Other visitors would demonstrate creative visualization, and we had, of course, Annette, who was great at leading visualizations. We also discussed vitamin and mineral supplementation. Our discussions included everything that was alternative in character, even color therapy.

Prior to my illness, I had already begun studying books like *Life and Teachings of the Masters of the Far East* by Baird T. Spalding. I went to a woman called Rhea Powell whom I call my spiritual awakener. I was already doing visualization, meditation, etc. So, for me, the group studies were not new, but a continued development along my own path.

There was also Tony Smith's group, The Great Pretenders. Its purpose is to do something for men in today's world. When I began attending their meetings, they had started a project to work with PWA's. Only three of us started with Tony. Although his group did not necessarily use the work of Louise Hay, it was suggested that we read her books. This group had a powerful effect on me. It was not exactly that they were more caring—there was much love in all of these groups—but they were more direct. There was no game-playing. We discussed the whole picture of AIDS.

We were committed to meet for three months, after which we would evaluate our progress and determine how we wanted to proceed. I realize more and more every day that what I received from them was wonderful. Yet, I didn't want to continue. Often, we can see more clearly, or appreciate more, in looking back than when something is happening.

Tony Smith wanted us all to go and experience Neuro-Linguistic Programming with Tony Robbins. I couldn't afford the entire weekend, but I agreed to go for the Friday and Monday night sessions at which we were shown videos on health and nutrition.

The Friday night session culminated in a fire walk. I can't fully describe what that did for me—doing the fire walk and just realizing what I had done! I walked across the fiery coals. It was such an achievement for me. Anything was possible! I could do anything! It was as if I could do the impossible—as if I already had!

In addition to the group support, certain books gave me hope and courage. I didn't study the *Course in Miracles*, but I read *Getting Well Again; Love Your Disease, It's Keeping You Well; Conquering AIDS Now!; Anatomy of An Illness;* and *You Can Heal Your Life.* All of these seemed directed toward me and my healing. A book that particularly inspired me was *Initiation* by Elisabeth Haich. Then there was Bach's *The Adventures of a Reluctant Messiah.*[1] When selecting something to study, I simply go down to any of the bookstores in this city and buy whatever seems to jump into my hand. My whole life now seems to be in a pattern of receiving things of meaningful help.

I monitor information. I do not believe everything I read in the newspapers and magazines, or what I hear on television. The media are very negative. I don't need negativity in my life at this time.

My spiritual life has taken on a definite ritual or pattern. I meditate every morning. I also channel, vocally through the mouth, and I channel on the piano. There is some great music for channeling. I go to a meditation group every Friday night in Manhattan, which is led by various people, such as Richard Brinckman. Also, Canning comes to New York once a month from California.

These are all channels, basically through Rhea Powers. Canning was Rhea's spiritual awakener. Rhea has traveled all over the world and Richard does her work in New York while she travels. There's a group of us who get together once a week for channeling.

Alternative therapies have helped me considerably. Actually, I decided that medical treatment was not, or would

---

[1]   See Bibliography at the end of this book.

not be, the treatment for me, even before I was diagnosed as a PWA.

I had—and still have—the feeling that AIDS is going to assist the whole world in understanding natural, alternative ways of healing. This does not negate the benefit I have received from the scientific world or what it is doing, because I'm in a balanced state between the two. I'm on AZT. I take a lecithin product once a day. I feel that I myself took control of my illness and its treatment.

Health improvement was slow. I had pneumocystis three times, but each time it was less severe than the preceding bout. The first time I was in the hospital for about four weeks, the second time for about ten days, and the last time for about seven days.

Although improvement was gradual, it was definite. Alternative therapies help you to listen to your body. I seemed to hear voices telling me that I was in the process of becoming well. According to my friends, I look better now than ever before.

I have grown very much through this illness, through the process of healing myself and the support of my friends and groups. I feel that I have blossomed. I keep coming up with that phrase. I don't know a better way to describe the difference I feel in myself, the uplifted feeling. I've opened up and am able to communicate almost everything that is blossoming within me.

As to my vulnerability to AIDS, I don't negate it. I've been diagnosed, and there's still much pressure from the outside, saying that it's going to be devastating for me. But right now, I feel healthy.

There is nothing exceptional in this feeling of wellness. The road to health is available to everyone. The essential thing is that each finds his own path. I feel that there is much more information to be received, and more of it must get out to the people. There is a vast void in the general population—a great ignorance of natural and spiritual therapies.

Those who do not survive AIDS are not necessarily doing anything wrong. On the deepest level, it is their decision. What went on previously in their lives to result in AIDS may be the basis for the decision. It is neither right nor wrong. It is simply their decision and they have the right to make it.

Just as the elements of your life lead up to a situation such as being diagnosed with AIDS, so these same elements, in a sense, contain the solution to this problem in your life. I moved out of my roommate situation, and now have my own apartment. I have developed a relationship with another man, who is incredible. Our relationship keeps growing. It's not like anything I've ever felt before. That sounds corny, I know, but it's true. I think anyone who has undergone what I'm describing understands what I mean.

When your life is going right, other things fall into place. My growth within my company has been marked. My boss remarks on my improvement in attitude.

These changes in my life are responses to my own change of thinking. In the past, I was a bit hard on myself and had a poor self-image. Now, I think I'm wonderful.

We get involved with life in general and we don't stop to consider our own lives. My illness forced me to look at myself and what I was doing. I really had to stop and evaluate my own mental processes and feelings. I had to get in touch with all that was going on inside me. I learned to understand that what I may have labeled as bad, is simply human nature. I don't, therefore, have to beat myself up for feeling like a human being. The answer is to work through your feelings, experience them and move on.

People often say, "When you're ready for love, somebody will come along, and you'll fall in love." I consider disease to be similar. I believe the universe acts like that. People look on illness as totally negative. But for me, it meant progress. Once we're prepared for something, we'll bring it into our lives.

I feel it is very important for an AIDS patient to hold onto the positive things, and not dwell on the gloom and doom presented in newspapers, television, radio, magazines, etc. There are people who are getting well. There is much new knowledge about the illness—but the media are not covering it. A whole new field of learning is opening up.

Find the books and movies that are inspiring, like the movie *Resurrection*. Many things not specifically directed at the disease can benefit you. It is important for the person to open up and get in touch with what is right for him or her. Some people feel that a macrobiotic diet is best. I started reading one of Michio Kushi's books on the subject and discovered that macrobiotics is more than a mere diet. The author lists some major problems on earth. One is divorce, another is homosexuality. I got that far in the book and closed it. I thought, "This author's attitudes are not for me."

A person should stay involved with life and not give up. He should listen to his body, to his mind, and spirit. The answer is there, whether it's life or death.

My former diet was the usual American food: meat, vegetables, dairy products, breads, salads. I still consume dairy products, but I rarely eat meat, fish, or poultry. There have been formal dinners I've had to attend where the entree was chicken. If I didn't eat that, I would go hungry. So, I'm not as strict with my diet as I was when I got started. I eat steamed broccoli, raw carrots, whole grains, and I drink fresh fruit and vegetable juices, but I still love cheese, and I really can't do without ice cream in the summertime. I allow myself to celebrate occasionally on birthdays, have a little champagne on New Year's—things like that. It was difficult finding all those health foods and making those changes. As I've gone along I've become a bit more relaxed in my choice of foods.

I am earning my living now designing women's clothing, working for a major firm in New York. But I still have dreams for the future. I have always dreamt of having my own design firm, putting my name on the labels, or perhaps being the design director for another company. I have always had dreams, and I still plan to make them a reality. I find another creative outlet in making most of my own clothes.

Spiritual creativity is the channeling I do on the piano. I don't know how to write music, but I would love to have someone transcribe it and perhaps even have some of it orchestrated.

Having had AIDS has broadened my spiritual concepts, but I have always felt close to God. I was brought up a Protestant, (United Church of Christ Congregational), but I have my own beliefs and understandings. I've never felt punished by God at all. Now I feel more at ease with people. I'm not afraid to let them see the "whole me" as I really am. I'm more direct and feel freer to assist friends in whatever problem or nonsense they're going through. My insight has greater depth and I am able to get to the heart of things. Part of my healing is passing on whatever I've learned.

When we heal an illness with natural and spiritual therapies, we are essentially healing our life.

"Fear is the fountain of sickness," wrote a great metaphysician. It is highly important, in the healing process, for the patient to rid himself of fear, and *replace this negative emotion with faith and understanding.*

WHAT "BERTIE CHAPIN" DID

- He realized that two or more opinions concerning diagnoses can exist at one time and that medical diagnoses are not 100% accurate.

- He was not overly worried about the AIDS diagnosis, but primarily concerned with curing his pneumonia.

- He had support from friends and groups. He became involved with the Well-Being Group in New York, whose purpose is to awaken the participants' personal powers, recognizing alternative types of healing and cultivating spiritual awareness.

- The group showed him that he wasn't alone, and that there were alternatives to allopathic medicine. Members of the group discussed the use of meditation, relaxation, visualization, channeling, nutrition (especially macrobiotic), acupuncture, supplementation, color therapy, etc.

- Natural therapies and spiritual paths helped him to listen to his body and to heal himself.

- He joined "The Great Pretenders," a group of men in New York City. They use Neuro-Linguistic Programming.

- He was a reader, and derived inspiration from the ideas in books.

- He did not believe everything he heard or read in the media. He protected himself from negative suggestions.

- He meditated every morning.

• He had decided, even before diagnosis, that he would not use harmful medical treatments, as he had seen so many friends die in hospitals under orthodox treatments for AIDS.

• He was willing to be patient for his healing.

• He took control of his living situation.

• He developed new relationships that kept him growing.

• His attitudes changed and his self-esteem and self-love grew.

• His disease broadened his spiritual concepts.

• People look on illness as totally negative—to be feared and avoided. But for him, it meant progress.

• "Bertie Chapin" believes that when we heal our illness, we heal our lives, and that each one must seek out his own paths.

"Paul Michael Allen"

Fasting is a therapy used in the natural health field with success, but not by orthodox medical practitioners. It has a long history, is used much in Europe and elsewhere abroad and has a large literature.

It is most important to emphasize that fasting does not mean starving the body. In fasting, a complete rest is given the body, including the digestive organs, so it can restore itself. Aging and sick cells are renewed; excess fat and abnormal deposits are absorbed, but the tissues and cells of vital organs are preserved. In starvation, this is not the case. The body ingests its vital tissues in order to sustain life. Starvation is dangerous to life, as we see in African countries where famine conditions prevail.

Fasting is not recommended in all AIDS cases. If a great weight loss has occurred and the body is emaciated, it is not recommended. However, in the following case study, the patient was overweight and success was achieved. If the patient has an advanced case of AIDS and has lost much weight, he should not fast but go on the diet plan described by the authors of the book *Conquering AIDS Now!*

A fast must be supervised by an expert, preferably in a fasting institution. Drugs should not be used during a fast, and the person should have plenty of water, rest, fresh air, sunshine, and a quiet mind, free from fear. The majority of humanity is so accustomed to three meals every day that it cannot imagine not eating for a week or two, and will be terrified to death, in its ignorance of the great therapeutic value of fasting.

Dr. Paavo Airola, prominent natural health doctor, recommended juice fasts instead of complete fasts (meaning no food at all, only water). He is author of *How to Keep Slim, Healthy and Young with Juice Fasting.*

Note that Russell John Carlton, whose story is in this book, used the juice fasting therapy under supervision with good success. He used carrot juice and herbs.

Here is a detailed report of a case of AIDS by Dr. Ralph C. Cinque, D.C., a chiropractor. He is Director of the Hygeia Health Retreat (a live-in facility offering fasting and nutritional programs for weight loss and health improvement), in Yorktown, Texas. Dr. Cinque has sent us the following report:

"'Paul Michael Allen' from New York City, 29, admittedly homosexual, had developed abdominal pain, frequent diarrhea, swollen cervical (neck) lymph nodes, intermittent fevers, rapid weight loss and severe weakness. He entered a hospital for tests and was told that the physicians thought he had AIDS. They wanted to keep him there for further testing and treatment, but he became afraid and checked out.

"A friend who knew about Natural Hygiene (this refers to a philosophy and practice where only natural methods and a vegetarian diet are used in healing) urged him to consider fasting, and made arrangements for him to come to our retreat. When he arrived, we fed him a Natural Hygiene diet for a day, and it was agreed that he would begin fasting on the second day. I explained to him that I had no way of knowing whether or not he had AIDS, but that we would treat him like anyone else, and be guided by his symptoms and progress.

"He fasted for fourteen days, during which time he experienced no crises, and only the expected amount of weakness and weight loss. By the end of the fast his abdomen was comfortable, his neck swelling had subsided, and his temperature was normal.

"We began feeding him Hygienically and he promptly began gaining weight and strength. After a week of eating he was ready to go home, and on his last night he put on a musical concert, playing the guitar and singing. He appeared to have abundant energy and complete physical and mental comfort. Although I have not heard from him since, I have every reason to believe that he has remained well."

[The authors of this book disclaim all responsibility in any case where a reader-patient tries fasting in a self-healing program.]

John Hampton

John Hampton, 30, of Los Angeles, says:
"I decided I wanted to heal myself and not use drugs. The people I've seen who are doing well are not doing it with drugs."

He was diagnosed with AIDS in July, 1987. He is now a leader of Mastery group sessions. More than 1,000 people have attended the sessions in Los Angeles, San Francisco, New York, Chicago, and Dallas. Such weekends have also been held in London, and Edinburgh, Scotland.

Hampton says: "I had been in a lot of denial, pretending I didn't have the disease. With the Mastery I went from denial to totally accepting the disease, but deciding I wanted to heal myself. There is so much support and such a loving group of people in the workshops. A great deal of spiritual work is done there."

He is on a strict nutritional diet, works out at a gym and swims an hour each day. "I do visualization and meditation every day, too. The only thing we really have control of in this life is our thoughts."

He also says he has read everything he can find about alternative cures,—"what's out there about AIDS. That's the first thing I tell people to do—get their hands on everything they can and read and decide what they want to pursue."

From *Los Angeles Times*, August 16, 1987

"J. H."

"It has been two years since my diagnosis of AIDS and I am proud to say that, thanks to alternative health and mental care, I am healthier, more productive and successful in my work, happier and more spiritually fulfilled than at any other time in my life.

"Each one must find his separate truths—and sharing of those truths with each other can only lead to a more profound understanding, awareness, and healing.

"There were many spiritual and physical choices I've had to make. They have caused my Kaposi's sarcoma to disappear, my energy to swell and my mind to begin to soar into a new realm of what can be."

J. H., Chicago, IL
(*Healing AIDS* newsletter, San Francisco

"Wood"

This information was received from "The Backroom," a gay computer resource in New York.

"'Wood', the nickname the survivor uses, had AIDS eight years ago in San Francisco. It was full-flowering, florid: PCP, KS—everthing on the list except the dementia. The disease had not progressed that far. He decided to stop all the hospital stuff, and go to a Mexican jungle to follow a man doing alternative medicine, like the kind described in *Conquering AIDS Now!* Wood recently breezed in and out of New York, doing TV interviews. Most of all he wanted to get out of the city and back to his jungle. But I hear he still maintains an apartment in San Francisco.

"He's the most healthy and alive person I've ever met."

"The Upper Westsider"
A Gay Computer Resource
(Voice) (718) 849-3335
(Modem) (718) 849-6699

"Charles Stevens"

A HEALING OF AIDS WITH CHRISTIAN SCIENCE

A young man who was an AIDS patient, near death in a New York City hospital, called a Christian Science church for help. (He had attended a Christian Science Sunday School years before, and a mental seed sowed then had sprouted in his consciousness, in his great hour of need. He had remembered and reached out, grasping at this last hope of life.)

A practitioner of the church responded immediately, and visited him in the hospital. The Lesson-Sermon for the week was on the subject "Sacrament," and the Christian Science practitioner read it aloud to the patient, at his bedside. At the end of the reading, the young man humbly asked to be helped out of bed so that he could kneel beside the bed and pray.

The practitioner was informed by the doctor that there was no need to come the next day—that the patient would most certainly be dead by then.

But the practitioner *did* visit the patient, and went to him daily for 48 days. He read to him from the Christian Science textbook (*Science and Health with Key to the Scriptures* by Mary Baker Eddy), and prayed with him. At the end of that time, the patient was pronounced completely healed and recovered, and left the hospital.

OTHER CHRISTIAN SCIENCE HEALINGS

Mr. Kentner Scott, President of Emergence International, has given us the following report. Emergence is a group of Christian Scientists supporting gay and lesbian people, and its address is: P. O. Box 581, Kentfield, CA 94914-0581.

Mr. Scott said that a Christian Science practitioner in New York had sent him the following letter, in her own handwriting:

"In my practice I have had many cases involving AIDS. I call to mind about ten of them. One was healed through Christian Science treatment even after he was hospitalized and four doctors confirmed the diagnosis of AIDS.

"This healing was more than three years ago. The man in the case has gone on to Christian Science class instruction, and has now started on a career as a practitioner. Another case was not so far advanced, but glandular swelling was deflated in one day after my treatment, and the symptoms have never returned.

"A third case was in a hospital four different times, and then rallied with a steadily-increasing T-cell count, to a point where he now lives a healthy, normal life."

———————

David James Nolan, of the Committee of United Christian Scientists (P.O. Box 8048, San Jose, CA 95125), has said of *They Conquered AIDS!*, "This book is throwing a lifeline to beleaguered humanity."

———————

Further help for Persons with AIDS, including a free booklet *Healing AIDS—The Action of Omnipotent Mind— a Christian Science Treatment* is available from ONE MIND, P.O. Box 6008, Washington, DC 20005-0708. If the writer gives his telephone number, he will be called with an offer of more assistance, and a loan copy of the book *Science and Health with Key to the Scriptures* by Mary Baker Eddy.

PART II

COMMENTARIES

AUTHORS' COMMENTS

ABOUT SURVIVORS

AIDS UPDATE

WHY WE CREATED THIS BOOK

(PART I — by Scott J. Gregory)

Our first book on AIDS, *CONQUERING AIDS NOW! With Natural Therapies, a Non-Drug Approach,* was the FIRST BOOK PUBLISHED to offer information on natural healing in connection with AIDS.

Readers would ask: "Where is your proof? If Holistic Healing really works, where are the 'recoverees'?" Those questions caused us to create *this* book.

The first book contains the *information*; this sequel contains the *demonstration*.

I studied the subject of Natural Healing in the early 1980's, in the U.S. and abroad. Intuition and inspiration also evoked a message to me that all mankind is naturally empowered with health. The path of harmony and balance is not outside of the individual; natural healing is from within outward. One cannot *drug* a body into health, or force an individual to believe that something will either harm him or benefit him. This applies to both allopathic medicine and the holistic philosophy.

As a health practitioner, I educate the individual and then let him decide on the mode of therapy he desires or feels an affinity for. We all need to develop our intuition.

Example: At age fifteen, I was diagnosed as having a staphylococcus infection. The doctor told me that I must take antibiotics for an indefinite length of time. But after some weeks, I realized they were doing more harm than good. I continued to suffer; I was not improving, but feeling worse and worse. I asked my higher consciousness for an alternative. The message was: "Stop taking the drug; go to a health food store and you will find the answer." I felt drawn to the idea of chlorophyll as my helper. At that time, few health food stores had chlorophyll, but I found it. I fasted from solid foods; I drank chlorophyll. A vegetable juicer was given to me, and I made fresh vegetable juices from green leafy vegetables. The "staph" infection vanished after a couple of days.

In the early 1980's, I worked as a nutritional consultant in a health food store. Persons with AIDS came to me for help. Empathically, I asked myself: "What can be done?" I received answers—not from books, not from doctors, not from past knowledge—but from intuition. I helped these individuals with their problem, and they recovered. This is how the first book, *CONQUERING AIDS NOW!* was born. Meeting Bianca Leonardo, a health author and publisher, made it possible.

I came from a long line of "sickies." I knew none of my grandparents; people on both sides of my family had all the serious diseases—cancer, diabetes, arthritis, and heart trouble. Most of my relatives died of chronic degenerative diseases. I am convinced that they suffered from a lack of health knowledge. They were ignorant of correct nutrition, and lacked harmony with the universe. In my family, I became the exception. From an early age, I taught myself prevention, nutrition, and self-care.

If an individual is looking for health, he should go to one who is practicing or demonstrating it—a healthy physician. Medical doctors are not health oriented; they are disease oriented. And that is one of the main problems with medicine today. Health practitioners should teach prevention, so that people do not get sick in the first place!

My Number One message to the AIDS patient is: "If you look hard enough for something, you will find it, whatever it is—good or bad, disease or health."

My Number Two message is: There should be no guilt on the part of the patient, and no condemnation or judgment of the ill person.

I am reminded of a childhood experience in Detroit. Both my parents worked. I was an only child—six years old at the time. After school, I was tended at the home of a Polish family. The baby sitters cooked Polish sausages for me; I would eat them, but always vomit on the floor.

The sitters were furious at me; they beat me, verbally and physically, and said that I was a bad boy. I thought: "How can I possibly be punished for something that *they* did to me?" I vowed that I would never judge or condemn anyone for being sick.

Persons with AIDS are not bad; they are ill. Let us not judge them and add to their burden.

Many of our Conquerors had to learn to dissolve self-blame and low self-esteem and see themselves in a higher light in order to recover.

How did we find our Conquerors? Some found our first book, and then found us. We advertised for survivors; we inquired of AIDS organizations; a few came "out of the blue." If something is in your consciousness constantly, this thought will empower the law of attraction. We sought, we asked, and we found—our Conquerors. We also sought and found the natural remedies in our books.

It is most significant that this book was conceived and largely written at a time when the whole world was saying that "AIDS is 100% fatal." Now we present the proof to the whole world that AIDS is *not* invariably fatal. A different approach must be taken from the traditional drugging one.

Freedom to make your own choices in health matters is your birthright. Claim it! It is already yours.

WHY WE CREATED THIS BOOK

(Part II — by Bianca Leonardo)

From childhood, I have felt a passion for life—and a compassion for mankind. Since its inception, this book has been "Dedicated to Suffering Humanity."

AIDS is claiming more and more victims, because of a lack of true health knowledge. Much heart-rending news of individual suffering is being called to our attention.

A young woman named Connie, five months pregnant, desires her baby very much. But she has tested HIV positive, and is being urged by her doctor to abort the baby. At this late stage, abortion is a lengthy process that takes three days. For two days the doctors proceed to kill the fetus; on the third day, they vacuum out the mass of death.

Connie is being advised that if she persists in bringing the baby to birth, a dire future lies in wait for herself and the infant. In despair, she is torn between two hard choices. Connie is not being advised of the danger to her health and life from an abortion at five months, or of the psychic damage of destroying the babe in her womb who is so near birth.

I feel compassion for Connie and innumerable others, known and unknown to me. Young men, older men, women and children—all suffering needlessly and dying prematurely. This love for humanity was my motivation for seeking out the truth about AIDS and all health problems.

Self-education and life experiences brought me to the point of a strong desire to create this book. Especially, there was a disillusionment with material medicine, as a result of seeing loved ones die prematurely and tragically in hospitals— sometimes from medical errors, always from the prevailing medical treatment. I suspect that today most Americans have such sad life experiences.

These are behind the great increase in medical malpractice suits.

At the age of 19, I was introduced to Christian Science by a friend. I immediately saw it as the truth about Life—about God and Man. The friend said that in my questions and his answers, I was "like a thirsty sponge." I had found a teaching that brought me joy, healing, and a deep understanding of what life really means and can be.

About 1970, I found the holistic health philosophy. It seemed to be like the missing part of a puzzle. I saw that it is illegitimate for one to abuse the body (even eating unhealthful foods is abusing the body), and then expect God to heal him. Our bodies are a trust to care for, with wisdom and understanding.

I did a great deal of reading, attended health conferences, and took courses at holistic health institutions—The Life Science Institute (Austin, TX) and the American Nutritional Medical Association (Colorado Springs, CO).

Both Spiritual Science and Holistic Health have a twofold nature: prophylactic (preventive) and therapeutic (having healing powers.)

Holistic living has many aspects, and is most individual. For me, it is a knowledge of nutrition, a vegetarian diet, and pure living. All my life I have been fortunate in never having any need or desire for drugs, alcohol, tobacco, coffee, etc.

Those who are very energetic must watch "overdoing," as that can cause stress. Planned, quiet times of meditation can help alleviate or even heal this tendency. Enthusiasm (from "en-theos"—God), is a marvelous quality. But it needs to be tempered by a still strength and serenity. Tempered zeal makes the world move.

Holistic Health principles work. I have experienced them myself and have seen them work in other lives. Holistic Healing can be applied successfully to AIDS, as our Conquerors show.

The holistic (wholistic) philosophy *does not mean* including every modality, such as material medicine. It *does mean* including the totality of body/mind/spirit; using *no* drugs of any kind; nutrition; the principle of moderation, especially in eating; right thinking and pure living, and other natural principles.

I am convinced that the spiritual is the highest form of healing, and is the wave of the future. It does not use the human mind as a remedial agent, but the divine Mind, or God. It is a vast subject. Some introductory hints on spiritual healing are given in this book you are reading.

*　　　*　　　*　　　*　　　*

I consecrate my life, my love, and my courageous endeavors toward alleviating the suffering of humanity. There is no greater work. May others find the joy of unselfed lives, and join in this holy cause.

—Bianca Leonardo

As I see it, the first goal for Natural Healing is achieving an amendment to the U. S. Constitution that will give it full powers, along with allopathy—as I have written elsewhere in this book.

The second goal will come more easily—the establishment of colleges where Natural Therapies can be taught, where healers can be trained. "Naturopathy" means the treatment of ailments with natural methods.

As of now, there are two colleges of Naturopathy in the U. S.— the National College of Naturopathic Medicine, 11231 S.E. Market St., Portland, OR 97216, and the Bastyr College, 144 N.E. 54th St., Seattle, WA 98105.

As of 1988, Arizona, Connecticut, D.C., Florida, Hawaii, Nevada, Oregon, Washington, and several provinces in Canada, permit graduates with the N.D. degree to practice with full rights. In other states the N.D. graduates must find a niche with another licensed doctor, or in some holistic setting.

There is a long way to go!

THE IMPORTANCE OF A CORRECT DIAGNOSIS
by Dr. Scott J. Gregory

It is most important for a patient to receive an accurate diagnosis. To diagnose a person merely by symptoms or clinical laboratory tests is flagrantly erroneous. Because one's immune system is suppressed does not necessarily mean that he has AIDS. Individuals who have some AIDS-like symptoms could be suffering from diseases other than AIDS.

CASE I: Here is a typical example of an erroneous diagnosis: "T.C." had no apparent exposure to AIDS but felt ill. He went to his doctor for testing, and after an HIV confirmation, the doctor informed him that he had been exposed to AIDS. "T.C." asked to have the two tests repeated, and both results were negative. What happened? He questioned the doctor, who replied that the laboratory had made a mistake. But the laboratory said that the doctor had not interpreted the results accurately. (HIV does not always appear in the blood.)

These tests are not given prior to AIDS or suspected AIDS. They are always given after a person has the signs and symptoms. (Signs are what one sees; symptoms could be within, or invisible, such as fatigue.) So, how does one know if he was or was not immuno-suppressed before the symptoms occurred? Conclusion: too much emphasis is placed on testing.

CASE II: Young "J.S.P." showed no signs or symptoms of AIDS. But he went to his doctor and took the standardized tests—the ELISA, the Western Blot, and the T-cell ratio subset. His doctor informed him that he was immuno-suppressed, and was suffering from AIDS. "J. S. P." told his friend Dr. Gregory:

"I've got to do something about my T-cells. The doctor says they are very low." Dr. G. replied: "How do you know they are low? What were they before this AIDS diagnosis?"

"J. S. P." replied: "I don't know. I never had them tested before."

Dr. G.: "Is it not possible that some individuals are born with low T-cells or they are immuno-suppressed <u>before</u>

AIDS?"

People are different in many ways. Some individuals have a proclivity toward immuno-suppression even prior to getting the disease. No serious disease comes "like a thief in the night"—suddenly.

Later, with full medical coverage from the V.A., "J.S.P." decided he would have a full set of lung X-rays. He was concerned that he would develop pneumocystis pneumonia (PCP). His doctor knew he was HIV positive and proceeded to do the chest X-ray. A couple of days later he received a report from his medical doctor stating there was some discoloration on the right lobe of his lung. Prior to that he had had no physical symptoms.

After receiving the report, "J.S.P." telephoned Dr. Gregory, stating that he had dyspnea, (difficulty in breathing), shortness of breath, and pain in the chest upon exertion. At that point Dr. G. told him the doctor should retake the X-ray. He called his doctor at the V.A.; they suggested he have a bronchoscopy. This test is the only true confirmatory test.

As a bronchoscopy is considered a major surgery, it was requested the X-rays be repeated. "J. S. P." called Dr. G., very much excited, saying the X-ray showed nothing there. Because of his fear of PCP, "J. S. P." had manifested the symptoms. This shows that the power of the mind is very important.

CASE III: "F.C." has a medical background, with doctors in his family. He had the signs and symptoms of AIDS; he had a gay lifestyle; his tests showed "positive." For all these reasons, the diagnosis of AIDS was a valid one. Only drugs were being offered by orthodox medicine, with no hope of healing foreseen. He developed pneumocystis pneumonia (PCP).

"F.C." had a great deal of money, and could do as he wanted concerning treatments. He decided that he wanted to use alternative therapies, and embarked upon a healing program. But in a short time, his symptoms became more serious. He dropped the natural therapies and returned to the hospital.

The medical family had put pressure on him to return to the medical ways. IV drugs were given for the AIDS. While in the hospital, he also ate junk food sweets that members of his family brought to him.

It takes time for the body to heal itself using natural therapies, but many individuals will not give the body the time it needs or trust these therapies. Conclusion: Natural Medicine is often abandoned because results are not immediately measurable.

DR. SCOTT J. GREGORY'S PROTOCOL
FOR AIDS/ARC, USING NATURAL TREATMENTS

Categories of Treatment and Suggested Natural Products

I. TO KILL THE VIRUS: powerful, non-toxic, harmless anti-viral agents are used.
    A. DIOXYCHLOR. Homeopathic tincture. Kills pathogenic microbes. Inorganic oxidant has been found to be effective against Candida Albicans and the AIDS virus (The Bradford Institute).
    B. LOMATIUM DISSECTUM TINCTURE. One of the most important widely-used American Indian remedies. In 1949, the sap of this herb was researched and made available. For coughs, asthma, pneumonia, tuberculosis, viral infections. It has been proved to kill harmful organisms, and inhibits the growth of various strains of bacteria. No toxic effects.
    C. OXYQUINOLINE SULPHATE. Homeopathic preparation. (Its original intention was for staphylococcus infection.)
    D. EXITOX (Smithsonite). A cationic solution (concerns the equilibrium of the cell) formulated in the 1800's by a world-famous German scientist. Known for its healing properties and recognized for its importance involving the immune response. It contains minerals and trace minerals that interact with enzymes. It supplies oxygen to the cells, purifying the blood and helping the body to overcome disease.
    E. MONOLAUREN (derived from mother's milk.)
    F. HYDROGEN PEROXIDE (H_2O_2)—Food Grade.
II. TO DETOXIFY AND RID THE BODY OF METABOLIC WASTES:
    A. DMG PLUS. (VITAMIN B-15 PLUS TMG—Tri-Methylglycine.) Oxygenates the blood, rids the body of uric acid, detoxifies the body of wastes.

    B. PHYTOBIOTIC HERBAL FORMULA, especially good for parasitic infections—*E. coli, giardia, cryptosporidum.*

    C. LIVA-TOX herbal preparation to help cleanse the liver

    D. Colonic or colemic intestinal irrigation

    E. Rectal feedings and implants with chlorophyll

    F. Saunas

    G. Clay Baths (Bentonite moss algae preferred)

    H. Mud baths

    I. Sulphur spring baths for Kaposi's sarcoma

III. TO ENERGIZE THE BODY:

    A. MEGA FOOD VITAMIN C, with Amino Acids and Minerals

    B. PROCAINE HYDROCHLORIDE GH-3

    C. OPTIMUM LIQUID MINERALS

    D. KM—Potassium Mineral Tonic

IV. TO BUILD THE IMMUNE SYSTEM:

    A. TARGET ZINC (Three kinds of zinc that target special organs)

    B. SHIITAKE MUSHROOM EXTRACT

    C. Raw Thymus

    D. Beta-Carotene

    E. Pure aloe vera juice

    F. Acupuncture

    G. Chinese Herbs

The T-Cells of some of Dr. Gregory's patients who have used these supplements have increased up to 50% in one week.

WATER: Water is the most important place to start the healing process since the body is over 60% water. Dr. Gregory recommends using distilled (if possible, distilled sterilized) water with pneumocystic-prone individuals. All other kinds of water (tap, spring, well water) have elements that are harmful for an immuno-suppressed system.

FOODS: Vegetables should be slightly steamed rather than eating them raw, because protozoans that live in the soil and cause pneumocystis are destroyed by heat.

Disclaimer

Dr. Gregory is <u>not</u> stating that the use of these products will cure AIDS. He is not prescribing or treating, but only suggesting. Information on the supplements in this section has been derived from the best professional sources. These products should be used with the guidance of a health professional.

If one prescribes for himself, it is his constitutional right, but the authors and the publisher assume no responsibility.

Dr. Scott Gregory is available for consultation.

His address is: P.O. Box 1222, Santa Monica, CA 90406

Drugs and Sorcery

Where are the majority of the people in the world looking for health?

In the prophetic last book in the Bible, Revelation, John in exile on the Isle of Patmos wrote:

"All nations are deceived by her sorceries."

And what is the meaning of 'sorceries'? The Greek word is "PHARMEKIA." The English root word "pharmacy" is derived therefrom as dealing with the dispensing of drugs. This is a sort of magic, sorcery or witchcraft. It is a modern superstition.

People of all nations have been deceived by the administration of these drugs. The people have been systematically induced to adopt the use of drugs, now the primary and most universally accepted mode designed for the amelioration of sickness and disease.

Drugs may cause a disappearance of symptoms (as they are suppressed or buried), but no true health! Actually, symptoms are nature's warning signals, and often cleansing processes.

"In vain shalt thou use many medicines, for thou shalt not be cured," said the prophet Jeremiah in the Old Testament.

So let us look to Nature—fresh air, sunshine, water (used internally and externally), natural foods, exercise, sleep and rest, and the last—positive mental attitude, joy, peace, friendliness, spiritual pursuits and practices, such as meditation and prayer. These are the seven essentials of health.

Many volumes have been written on the vegetarian way of life, on its healthfulness. But it has a tremendous significance for mankind*, far beyond diet. Books can sometimes guide seekers to vital truths they can learn in no other way.—B.L.

---

* See *Deep Thoughts on War and Peace and Other Essays on the Vegetarian Way of Life* by Bianca Leonardo.

LONG-TERM SURVIVORS
by Michael Callen

Michael Callen (PWA Coalition in New York) found these qualities in the 17 long-term survivors he interviewed.

1. All of them had dabbled in alternative approaches. With KS, there were several striking stories of success with macrobiotic or vegetarian diets. About half of the long-term survivors had made major diet changes. The rest paid more attention to their diets.

2. Most or all had used approaches such as shiatsu massage, acupuncture, or visualization. A clear majority were involved with groups such as Louise Hay, or AIDS Mastery or Metaphysical Alliance.

3. All but two found solace in religion—about half in the religion of their childhood. Others did not seek organized religion, but spoke of spirituality, or a sense of oneness. None became Bible-thumping fundamentalists. All who did become involved in churches were critical of some aspects of organized religion.

4. All said they needed hope to survive. Each had to deal in some way with the media's repeated message that everyone dies. Some found it important to know survivors; many knew each other. All but two are aggressively involved in the AIDS movement, or working with PWA's; many are in the forefront.

5. They are fighters, often difficult patients, not passive. Most used a group of physicians to coordinate their care, not just one. A majority have fired a physician, or

ordered one out of their hospital room.

6. Several had moving, near-death experiences.

7. There was no magic bullet, no single treatment used by all the survivors. Not all of them use lipids, or macrobiotics, or ribavirin, or anything else. Their experience suggests that AIDS is not one disease, with one substance that will work for everyone.

—From article "Not Everyone Dies of AIDS" in *The Village Voice*, New York City, May 3, 1988 (Vol. XXXIII, No. 18.) With permission of Michael Callen

*   *   *   *   *

Michael Callen was diagnosed six years ago with AIDS. He is a founding member of the People with AIDS Coalition in New York, and of the Community Research Initiative.

Community Research Initiative, Attn: Thomas Hannan, Administrative Director, c/o People with AIDS Coalition, 263A West 19th Street, Room 125, New York, New York 10011.

"C.R.I." is calling for a creative approach to AIDS research. Contributions are tax deductible.

Michel Callen is also a singer and songwriter with an album entitled *Purple Heart*; it is about his experience of "living with AIDS." Available from "Significant Other Records," P.O. Box 1545, Canal Street Sta., New York City 10013.

WHY SOME OF THOSE WHO HAVE CONQUERED
AIDS KEEP A LOW PROFILE

At a time when it is blasphemy to suggest that there is a cure for AIDS outside of an as-yet-undiscovered potent drug, when physicians won't even come to a public meeting where a successful self-treatment program is revealed, when communities are so unreasonably panicked by the specter of AIDS that they spawn people like the arsonists who burned the home of three children who have the disease, when initiatives are afloat to forcibly segregate infected individuals from their loved ones and communities of support—at a time like this, you don't have to ask twice why many who have survived AIDS past their expected lifespan have kept their good news to themselves.

Do you think I am exaggerating the situation? If physicians weren't afraid to appear to their colleagues as quacks or quack fellow-travelers, they would at this very moment be reading this book on natural, alternative therapies—*Conquering AIDS Now!* by Scott J. Gregory and Bianca Leonardo.... A quick look at the contents tells why it isn't on the desk of every doctor involved with AIDS. (She lists some of the natural therapies described in the book.)

"Surviving AIDS?", column,
"Health", *L. A. Weekly,* September 11-17, 1987.

SURVIVING AIDS?—PART 2

George Melton, who has been diagnosed with ARC, and Wil Garcia, who has been diagnosed with AIDS, are survivors. They've embarked on a national tour to spread their view that AIDS is not incurable.

Using meditation as their primary tool to pry within and discover the source of their illnesses, Melton and Garcia eventually managed to confront their inner demons and chase them away. Melton forced himself to recognize that self-hate was behind the suicide he was committing with his lifestyle. He saw that he'd allowed himself to be defined by his sexuality, as though that was all he had to offer. And he noticed that it had taken only a month for him to create an ulcer out of the stress of his ARC diagnosis. Once he focused his attention on the feelings behind the distress, his ulcer disappeared as quickly as it had come.

Garcia now believes that the link between our thoughts and our body is our emotions. When negative emotions arose, he tried to find the core of those feelings. A telling example, he says, is that if Melton spilled wine on a host's carpet, Garcia would feel terribly embarrassed and begin to apologize for Melton's clumsiness. Through the process of self-discovery, he began to ask what that embarrassment was all about. Was this sense of responsibility for the actions of others really necessary? Today, he says, he no longer allows himself to remain "on autopilot, getting upset" because of the actions of another.

For Garcia, the change in his T-cell count (from 25 in December of 1985 to between 800 and 900 today) is only one of the seeming miracles of healing that attending to his emotional life has initiated. For three years, he awoke with abdominal pain from chronic colitis. "His bedtable looked like a pharmacy," Melton recalls. However, "When he dealt with his feelings, his colitis went away as fast as my ulcer did."

In addition to using meditation and self-reflection, the

duo ate more simply and more naturally. They followed the "Fit for Life" diet, a controversial plan that includes a lot of fruit and vegetables, and little or no cooked foods or animal protein. ("I could do fruit for breakfast, cheat for lunch, and go back on the diet for dinner," jokes Garcia.) They do not advocate that everyone follow the exact same program, but advise others to choose nutritious foods and utilize physical therapies such as acupuncture, massage and chiropractic. Most important, they say, you should look within for the direction to go.

It isn't as difficult for us to change our beliefs as we may think, the men insist. All it takes is a reversal of the process that caused our automatic reactions in the first place: repetition. They recommend affirmations, which, simply put, are a repetition of a positive message to replace the old, negative ones unconsciously accepted from childhood. In a previous century, a favorite was, "Every day in every way I'm getting better and better."

Some may *not* be getting better, however, even with all this wonderful inner work. "There will be many people who do this work and still die, " admits Melton. Yet, he says, "Death isn't a failure. The issue isn't did I live or die, but what did I choose to do with the time I had?" Adds Garcia, "If our bodies don't heal but our soul does, that's a success."

At bottom, they advise, "Just because the doctor doesn't have the answer, that doesn't mean there isn't an answer. Look within!" From the 25 appearances they've already made, they can report with enthusiasm that more and more people are willing to follow their advice. Even in smaller Middle American communities, people are opening up to the possibility of healing themselves. "We act as a catalyst," Melton and Garcia proudly report.

"Because we come from such a scientific society, others have been afraid to believe that there was an answer that wasn't 'scientific,' " suggests Garcia. "The belief system in this country is, 'It's incurable.' "

    They call it "false fear," in contrast to what some may claim is the "false hope" of alternative therapies. "Hope, even false hope, allows you to take action," says Melton. "Without hope, constructive action isn't possible." With hope, the last laugh is theirs.

"Surviving AIDS? Part II", column,
"Health", *L. A. Weekly*, August 12-18, 1988.
Both articles by Carolyn Reuben.

The quoted item here was found to be incorrect.
It is therefore retracted and deleted by the publisher.

*   *   *   *   *

FLASH! BREAKTHROUGH ON AIDS
IN WEST GERMANY

This book, *They Conquered AIDS!* was going to the printer in a few days, when one of our Conquerors gave us this MOST SIGNIFICANT NEWS. Hold the presses—our readers must hear this!

Several dozen AIDS patients have not only reversed their death sentence, but are now back at work, completely free of the disease, in West Germany. They destroyed the virus in their blood by hyper-oxygenation (known in various forms as oxygen therapy, bio-oxidative therapy, or auto-hemotherapy).

The two basic types of oxygen therapy are ozone blood infusion, and absorption of oxygen water (hydrogen peroxide) at very low concentrations.

The Basis of Bio-Oxidative Therapies: Our bodies are composed mostly of water, which is 8/9 oxygen. Most nutritional studies get caught up in the small details of biochemistry and overlook our most abundant and essential element, and the fundamental role of its depletion in causing illness. Of all the elements the body needs, only oxygen is in such constant demand that its absence brings death in minutes.

Under conditions of optimum health, H_2O_2 is produced by the body's immune system. When the body is oxygen-starved, it can't produce enough H_2O_2 to wipe out the invading pathogens which cause visible disease.

If oxygenation is so simple and effective, why has it taken so long to discover it? Just exactly what would happen if a cure were discovered that is completely effective against the vast majority of diseases, ridiculously cheap and plentiful, and in most cases self-administered without a physician?

The complete report is available from:
Tree of Life Publications, 255 N. El Cielo Rd., #126, Palm Springs, CA 92262, for $5.00 postpaid.

AIDS AND THE ZEST FOR LIFE
by Ed Sibbett

(Courtesy, "Healing AIDS," newsletter, 3835—20th St., San Francisco, CA 94114.)

There are people who are HEALING THEMSELVES OF AIDS and other so-called incurable diseases. How is this possible? What do they know that we don't? Do they possess an uncommonly strong will to live? Could it be that they love life too much to give in to illness? Or perhaps they simply have more important things to do than to be consumed with sickness, dying and death.

It is important that each Person With AIDS takes a long, hard look at his life and asks: "How do I feel about myself in the context of the health crisis? Do I just *not want to die,* or do I *really want to live*?"

If you choose the latter, if you *really* want to live, you can! Start NOW to look for THE ZEST FOR LIFE.

What is the ZEST FOR LIFE? It's learning, growing, giving to myself and others, doing everything one can, following his dreams with love as his guide, and somewhere along the way the ZEST joins in. Each person will have to determine that magic balance of qualities and attitudes that works for him/her, but with patience, a loving outlook and commitment, we can and will find THE ZEST FOR LIFE.

At a conference of metaphysical leaders I attended recently, I spoke with Reverend Kennedy Schultz of the Atlanta Church of Religious Science. He told me that through working with the people in his AIDS healing group, he discovered that the ZEST FOR LIFE was the important element between those who got better and those who didn't. He said that it is the *key*, the *one* thing that makes all the difference; it is missing in those who do not get better. He went on to say that while most people *don't want to die,* not everyone *really wants to live,* to be a powerful part of the life force, to be in the positive energy of life. Further, he said that we must not allow ourselves to be brought down by negative forces and negative people who look upon us as dying, whether they're friends, relatives, the media or whoever or whatever. Don't give in to their ignorance and negativity.

Remember, we are not a passive entity; we are an active, dynamic life force. This is great news, because it is empowering. And empowerment is the whole point. It is very important that we don't give away our power by being passive. Accept the fact that you have the Power to add this key element to your life, this ZEST. Turn on that life force and start the healing where it really begins—within!

So, if you really want to live, do it. START NOW! Look for more and more exciting reasons and ways to enjoy life NOW, today...it is truly the only time we can ever do anything. Tomorrow is always the future and yesterday is only a memory. So watch out when you say things like: "I'll start tomorrow, or when I feel better, or have more money," or what's worse—"when they find a cure." These things are like a horizon—always out there, forever elusive. We are concerned with here and now. This very moment is the only time we will ever really have. So, NOW is the time for action, for doing, for healing, for LIFE and all the ZEST you can pack into it.

I ACCEPT MY POWER AND COMMIT MYSELF TO CHANGE. (Take these words and make them your own.)

I know that I am an active, *powerful* entity who exists in the *positive energy of the life force.* I therefore release all negativity that is blocking my healing—all fear, anger, resentment. And, as I release this negativity, I find that I have outgrown the need for illness—it has no hold on me now.

Grass Roots AIDS Organizations

In addition to state, county, and municipal departments and similar agencies, more than 3,000 grass-roots volunteer movements have sprung up since the epidemic began. The following are some of the larger non-profit organizations or groups.

Gay Men's Health Crisis
129 W. 20th St.
New York, New York 10011

American Foundation for AIDS Research
Box AIDS
New York, NY 10016

The AIDS Health Project
Box 0884
San Francisco, CA 94143-0884

The Kupona Network
4611 S. Ellis Ave.
Chicago, IL 60653

Shanti Project
525 Howard St.
San Francisco, CA 94105

Project Inform
347 Dolores St., Suite 301
San Francisco, CA 94110

AID Atlanta
1132 W. Peachtree St., N.W.
Atlanta, Georgia 30309

National Association of People With AIDS
2025 I St., N.W.
Washington, DC 20006

AIDS Foundation Houston
3927 Essex Lane
Houston, Texas 77027

Northern Lights Alternatives
78 W. 85th St., Suite 5E
New York, NY 10024

AIDS Project Los Angeles
3670 Wilshire Blvd., Suite 300
Los Angeles, CA 90010

ACT UP
496-A Hudson St., Suite G4
New York, NY 10014

AIDS Action Committee Boston
661 Boylston St., 4th Floor
Boston, MA 02116

Also, there is a toll-free AIDS hotline number for anyone with a question about AIDS. The number is 1-800-342-AIDS.

DR. BENJAMIN RUSH
and
FREEDOM OF HEALTH

Dr. Rush was a signer of the Declaration of Independence and the Surgeon General of the Continental Army. He was a physician who was a luminary that brought distinction to medical science. He left seeds of thought which, if acted upon by the profession, would have organized medical thought and prevented the present day confusion. Here are some of his wise comments on medicine:

"The whole *materia medica* is infected with the baneful consequences of the nomenclature of disease, for every article in it is pointed only against their names...By the rejection of the artificial arrangement of diseases, a revolution must follow in medicine.

"Humanity has likewise much to deplore from this paganism in medicine. The sword will probably be sheathed forever as an instrument of death, before physicians will cease to add to the mortality of mankind by prescribing for the names of diseases.

"The physician who can cure one disease by a knowledge of its principles may by the same means cure all the diseases of the human body, for their causes are the same.

"I am pursuing Truth, and while I can keep my eye fixed upon my guide, I am indifferent whither I am led, provided she is my leader."

On Health Freedoms

"We have provided for Religious and Political Freedom, but unless we make Provision for Medical Freedom, our best efforts to establish a Government of free men, shall prove abortive and the American people will ever be in bondage."

Dr. Benjamin Rush said this to the immortal mover of Freedom, Thomas Jefferson.

Dr. Rush urged the other founding fathers to include health freedoms in the Bill of Rights. It is a tragedy that his urgings were denied.

Did he foresee the future and our present medical monolith, as the monster it has become, and a monopoly at that, tolerating no other systems, although they be more humane, more scientific, and more effective in many cases?

Monopoly is illegal in other areas. Now it must be seen as erroneous and declared illegal in the field of health.

Both enlightened doctors who wish to use alternative-to-drug therapies and patients who want them also, are suffering from the tyrannical system. Dr. Benjamin Rush's prophecy has come true. The American people are in bondage in the field of health.

A NEW AMENDMENT TO THE CONSTITUTION OF THE U.S.
AN URGENT, DESPERATE NECESSITY

The people of the U.S. must demand—through their representatives—AN AMENDMENT TO THE CONSTITUTION. This will give U.S. citizens FREEDOM OF HEALTH—the freedom to choose any healing therapy desired, and doctors to use therapies other than drugging.

It is late, but not too late. Health freedoms for Americans were not established 200 years ago in our Constitution, but can be established TODAY, via an amendment to the Constitution!

What is needed: enlightenment of the people, and the people sufficiently caring, so they will insist to their representatives that the medical monopoly be stopped and FREEDOM OF HEALTH be granted instead—to doctors and the people alike. Let each person do something, no matter how small the act seems—to work toward this most worthy goal in America—FREEDOM OF HEALTH!

VACCINATIONS: MAKE THEM OPTIONAL

Barbara Loe Fisher is Executive Vice President of DIS-SATISFIED PARENTS TOGETHER (DPT), 128 Branch Road, Vienna, VA 22180. Phone (703) 938-3783. A kit for parents and a book entitled *DPT—A Shot in the Dark* , are available. Mrs. Fisher is co-author of the book. She writes:

We should have the right to make health-care decisions for ourselves and our children without interference from the state. Millions of parents are taking their children to doctors to receive seven vaccinations legally required for school. An unknown number will suffer severe reactions, become mentally retarded, paralyzed, epileptic, learning disabled, or even die, as a result of these vaccinations.

Every day, our organization hears from desperate mothers and fathers whose children aren't being allowed to attend school, who don't want their children injected with vaccines they consider unsafe. Some are being threatened with child-neglect charges.

Parents of children who have suffered severe reactions to the DPT shot too often can't find pediatricians to write medical exemptions so the children can attend school. Others are having physicians' exemptions rejected by state officials.

Zealous enforcement of vaccination laws is rooted in a 1904 Supreme Court decision that mandatory vaccination was justified because "medical men" could predict who would be harmed. The thousands of children killed or brain-injured by vaccines in the last 84 years are tangible proof that medical science is not infallible.

Drug companies race to develop a vaccine for AIDS; dozens of other vaccines are being created and targeted for mass, mandatory use. When health officials determined to achieve high vaccination rates and drug companies eager to realize high profits promote mandatory use, the public will be told about benefits, but rarely about risks.

In a nation with a tradition of valuing individual life, is there any justification for requiring parents to sacrifice their babies for society? (society's beliefs—Ed.) We shouldn't be forced to play vaccine roulette with our children; we should have the right to become educated about vaccines and make vaccination decisions without being threatened by anyone.

Authors' Note: Those parents who would like to avoid the current compulsory vaccination laws until they can be changed through political actions may wish to utilize the religious exemptions available. Write to Life Science, 6600-D Burleson Rd., Austin, TX 78760 (Ph 512-385-2781). Request membership in Life Science (which is free), and two copies of their exemption form.

When dealing with public officials you must be firm and realize that officials will often give you incorrect and misleading information. You must become informed and insist on your and your child's right against compulsory vaccination. Compulsory vaccination is a myth—you need not have your child vaccinated despite what misinformed teachers, administrators, or government officials may tell you. Many states have compulsory vaccination laws on the books, but all of these laws can be challenged and struck down with competent legal help and an effort to gain media attention for your cause. The religious exemption, however, will apply regardless of what state or city you live in.

How to Get Free Press by Delacorte, Kimsey, and Halas is an excellent book to utilize public support for your cause. And Nolo Press's self-help law books can help you in finding competent legal help in striking down local and state laws that are outdated and unenlightened. Write Nolo Press, 950 Parker St., Berkeley, CA 94710 or call 415-549-1976.

"THE REJUVENATION RETREAT"—
NATURAL THERAPIES HEALTH CENTER TO COME

("Rejuvenation" means, literally, "making young again.")

In material medicine, only the physical body is considered. Body, mind, and spirit are treated as one in holistic healing. A natural therapies health center or retreat is essential for this healing work.

The city environment, where most of the AIDS diagnoses and fatalities occur, is not conducive to health. Cities breed stress, noise, crime, fear, and pollution of the body and mind— all antagonistic to natural healing. Therefore, the ideal health retreat should be away from big cities.

When an AIDS crisis occurs, most persons don't know what to do or where to go. Of course, they see doctors. But they are frightened and confused. Weak and enervated physically, most PWAs are also in a mental state of doubt, depression and desperation. They are victims in the sense they cannot choose the type of health care they want. If they are inclined toward natural therapies, guidance and instruction are not easily available.

Those who are strong and knowledgeable say: "Here is the therapy I choose." Those who are weak and without health knowledge, say to friends, relatives and doctors: "Do whatever you will with me."

There will be a place. Those who seek natural therapies will find them. And they won't have to leave the United States.

THIS IDEAL HEALING RETREAT WILL BE REALIZED

- A place where people can truly get well, where the environment is conducive to healing.

- A place where people get encouragement instead of discouragement.
- A place of hope instead of despair—where people are told they will get well, not "you have only __ more weeks (months) to live."
- A place where a variety of natural modalities are combined that complement each other. Natural therapies are intensified in this way.
- A place where the sick are not judged, ridiculed, or blamed.
- A place where the sick are loved.
- A place where people are happy to be.
- A place where people can be educated in natural treatment, and where they can learn the true cause and prevention of disease, so that it does not occur again. They gain a knowledge of health for the remainder of their lives.
- A place where one is not a prisoner. A place where there is no fear of what someone is going to do to you, but where you choose your own therapies, with assistance. Where there is guidance and counseling. A place where you are in control, and can participate in your own healing.
- A place where "The Seven Essentials of Health" are used: Fresh Air, Pure Food, Sunshine, Water, Exercise, Rest and Sleep, and the Power of the Mental-Spiritual.
- A place where there are choices of food, and where healing herbs are used.
- A place that provides rest, relaxation, and peace of mind, and where there are options of solitude, prayer, and fasting.
- A place where people's concepts of healing can solidify and manifest.

- A place where people can be free from whatever interferes with their healing—persons, places, or things, or fears associated with them.
- A place where people can express themselves.
- A place where one can recapture playing.
- A place where not profits, but patients, are put first.
- A place that is financially stable, and able to help patients who can't afford treatment.
- A place where natural therapies are proven.
- A place where "whatever works" is used.
- A place where the practitioners and patients cooperate with Nature.
- A place where the practitioners might include: doctors of Oriental Medicine, using herbs, acupuncture, etc., chiropractors; naturopathic doctors; medical doctors who are trained in natural therapies or the New Medicine, and practitioners of various New Age modalities, such as hydrotherapists, homeopaths, and spiritual healers.

THE REJUVENATION RETREAT DESCRIBED

The environment is soothing.

The buildings are created around trees, brooks, etc., so that the man-made encompasses the natural. The architecture is influenced by the environment, as with Frank Lloyd Wright's or Japanese architecture.

Closeness to Nature is our ideal and goal, because we realize that Nature cooperates with the healing process.

The structures will be made of natural materials, such as wood, marble, stone, bamboo, and others, rather than chemicalized synthetics. Lighting is natural—full-spectrum. There will be nothing artificial to interfere with healing.

The site will be on grid-lines with the maximum electro-magnetic energy, conducive to healing. The site will be ecologically sound, with positive, rather than negative vibrations. The location will be near powerful negative ions. It must be near water: ocean, natural springs, or running waters such as brooks or rivers. Hot, bubbling, geothermic waters are very important.

Libations and Baths. Steam saunas with the healing waters. The water and the mud (hot springs coming through the earth) will be used for healing. Immersion in such mud is especially helpful in eliminating toxins.

The waters the guests will be drinking and bathing in will contain lithium, a naturally-occurring substance aiding mental health and states of well-being. It is found in some foods and certain waters.

Libations, for internal and external cleansing. Baths help to resolve mental and physical error and aid in spiritual experiences. The use of music. Certain musical notes have healing powers, and these will be used—especially played on lutes or other ancient instruments. (The sound of B flat is very healing.) Subliminal recordings will also be utilized.

Healing foods and juiced nectars will be prepared and served by godlike, spiritual individuals. Everyone at the retreat will be a healer. Those with power to heal with laying on of hands will be on the staff.

Circular (360°) solariums will be constructed with stained glass windows. These circular rooms will revolve. As they do so, the sun is directed through different colored panes of glass.

Aromatherapy will be used: the ancient art of healing through the sense of smell. The sense of smell has been shown to be a strongest link to memory experience. Certain aromas are associated with—anchored to—a time of well-being. We're creating a healing environment that makes people feel good.

There will be trained psychologists who are supportive and who suggest helpful ways to clear out thought forms destructive to the healing process. The word "psychology" comes from "psyche"—the soul. Our psychologists will be "soul workers." Lecturers will speak on different modalities of healing, so that the patient can decide what therapies are best for his body.

Laughter therapy, Reichian, Reiki, Gestalt, movement therapy, dance therapy, Rebirthing, Japanese Reality therapy, play therapy and pet therapy will be available—to be chosen by the patient.

There will be courses offered in Cooking for Health, Chinese medicine, Neuro-Linguistics, Electromagnetism, Ayurvedic Medicine, Body, Mind and Spirit Rejuvenation, Cooperation with Nature and Natural Healing—the New Medicine, and Spiritual Science.

The clinic will do work with electromagnetic phase conjugation resonance such as that used by R. B. Prior, a French scientist who cured cancer using electromagnetic resonance.

Guests will be taught how to turn off the negative mind through meditation, affirmations, visualizations, and the development of alpha and theta states.

To restore health, it is of primary importance to eliminate toxins and to re-establish physical, mental and emotional equilibrium. After health is restored, one can reach for a super-state in which the emphasis is no longer placed on physical healing, but an uplifting of consciousness—the mind, soul, and spirit. One no longer needs to be concerned about his body in this super-state of consciousness.

This innovative retreat is the authors' *ideal*. Let's make it *real*. It is a courageous goal that requires people, funding, and organization. Contact "Tree of Life Publications," and help make it happen.

*　　*　　*　　*　　*

DEEP THOUGHTS FROM GREAT MINDS
ON HEALTH

"A merry heart doeth good like a medicine."—King Solomon in Proverbs.

". . . it is not proper to cure the body without the soul."—Socrates.

"Most doctors err in their treatment. In endeavoring to assist nature, they weaken the body with their prescriptions."
—Maimonides, physician-philosopher.

"I'm not strong enough to stand the remedies; it's all I can do to stand the disease."—Moliere, French playwright.

"There is now incontrovertible evidence that mankind has just entered upon the greatest period of change the world has ever known. The ills from which we are suffering have had their seat in the very foundation of human thought."—Pierre Teilhard de Chardin, French philosopher and explorer.

"To ward off disease or recover health, man as a rule finds it easier to depend on healers than to attempt the more difficult task of living wisely."
—Rene Dubos, bacteriologist.

"The witch doctor succeeds for the same reason the rest of us succeed. Each patient has his own doctor within."
—Albert Schweitzer. From his autobiography *Out of My Life and Thought*.

"Instruct the sick that they are not helpless victims, for if they will only accept Truth, they can resist disease and ward it off, as positively as they can the temptation of sin. . . .The fact that Truth overcomes both disease and sin reassures depressed hope. It imparts a healthy stimulus to the body, and regulates the system. It increases or diminishes the action, as the case may require, better than any drug, alterative, or tonic. . . .

"Tell the sick that they can meet disease fearlessly, if they only realize that divine Love gives them all power over every physical action and condition."
—Mary Baker Eddy, in *Science and Health with Key to the Scriptures*, page 420.

THE VALUE OF BOOKS

BOOKS are the depositories of mankind's wisdom.

BOOKS are the most precious inventions of mankind.

BOOKS are the way discoveries and ideas of great men and women are carried on to future generations.

In the pages that follow, we share with you wisdom from a few significant books on topics related to this book. They can change your life.

Our aim is to help you stimulate your own research in this most vital area of knowledge—true health.

In these books you can learn the true cause of disease, the prevention of disease, and how to truly conquer disease.

Here are books that can open new doors for you—to a life of wisdom, a knowledge of how to care for your "temple."

These books can help you achieve a life free from suffering. They will enrich you, and health is true wealth.

—Bianca Leonardo

"A good book is the precious lifeblood of a master spirit, embalmed and treasured up on purpose to a life beyond life. Books contain a potency of life in them as active as that soul was whose progeny they are."

—Milton

"Books give new views to life, and teach us how to live."

—George Crabbe

"A good book is the purest essence of a human soul."

—Carlyle

"Books are the immortal mind of man."

—Author Unknown

WHY BOOK REVIEWS IN THIS BOOK?

These book reviews are being included here as a means of further educating the reader on some of the topics covered in this book.

ROGER'S RECOVERY FROM AIDS: How One Man Defeated the Dread Disease, by Bob Owens, 1987. Davar, P. O. Box 6310, Malibu, CA 90265

This interesting and important book is in the form of a novel. While one is reading *ROGER'S RECOVERY,* he wonders: is this true or fiction?

I, (B.L.) spoke with the author and he assured me: "All the people are real, but the names are fictitious. All the happenings are true."

This is the story of two friends, both medical doctors. One, "Roger Cochran," has contracted AIDS. After spending all his resources but getting no help from his own medical profession in this life crisis, he has nothing but death to look forward to. He visits the office of an old friend, "Dr. Bob Smith." They had known each other in Viet Nam. Dr. Smith at first does not recognize him—Roger is so emaciated. Roger asks his friend to help him, but Dr. Smith has no experience with AIDS. At first he cannot think of what he can do for his friend, but promises he will do whatever he can.

So begins an educational odyssey—the step-by-step self-education of Dr. Bob Smith. He discovers alternative, natural therapies. First he puts Roger on a change of diet (deleting his favorite food, steaks); then he puts Roger on a long fast. Bob Smith has accidentally come across books on fasting, and discovers new truths never learned in medical school. Because he has had no experience with fasting, either in his own life or with patients, both he and Roger are somewhat frightened. However, as no other options are at hand, the plunge is taken. *Roger recovers!*

A climax in Dr. Smith's self-education is while studying Dr. John Tilden's book *Toxemia—The Basic Cause of Disease.* Smith suddenly realizes: It isn't virus infection that Roger has. It's toxemia. It's uneliminated poisons!

The doctors involved declined using their true names, so they could continue their new work unhindered by publicity. They both are working in the healing art from this new standpoint.

The last chapter is called "A Word from Roger."

These vital quotations give the essence of the chapter:

"...Because of the persecution experienced by professionals who utilize non-toxic alternative health-care methods and procedures, many of these individuals, including Dr. Bob and myself, have tended to project a low profile, for their own economic, emotional and physical safety..."

"...we strongly recommend that, individually, or in concert with advocates of alternative health-care, you petition your political representatives to enact or amend laws which will make alternative options available.

"...if you wish to investigate some alternative treatment institutions and/or health-care professionals, it is your constitutional right to do so. To assist you in this endeavor, I suggest you contact Project CURE and the National Health Federation. Both organizations are actively engaged in keeping their constituents informed regarding orthodox medicine's self-serving attempts to pass laws limiting individuals from freely choosing their own health-care services. Both are also involved in enlisting the support of all interested U.S. citizens in preventing the passage of such laws.

Their addresses are:

Project CURE, 2020 K Street, N.W., Suite 350, Washington, D.C. 20069.

National Health Federation, 212 W. Foothill Blvd., Monrovia, CA 91016.

"These organizations are but two of the many groups that are working toward this cause, but they will give you a place to begin asking your questions. Furthermore, they will both help keep you informed concerning these vital issues as well as instruct you in getting actively involved in letter-writing campaigns that will make a difference.

"On a personal level, thanks to a doctor who was willing to put his practice and his future on the line for me, I am a well man today. Now we are working hard together to open the doors to alternative health care, so that other informed doctors won't run the risk of laying their futures on the line to freely treat their patients, and to make it possible for you to make your own personal health-care choice.

"We can't do this alone. We need your help. This you can do by contacting one or both of the agencies above and requesting information. Then, fully informed, begin contacting and airing your opinions with your state and federal representatives.

—Roger Cochran, M.D."

TOXEMIA, THE BASIC CAUSE OF DISEASE , John M. Tilden, M.D. Natural Hygiene Press, a division of The American Natural Hygiene Society, Inc., P.O. Box 30630, Tampa, FL 33630.

Dr. John Tilden was a sincere seeker after truth, honest and courageous. At his death at 89, he had practiced medicine 68 of those years, from 1872 to 1940.

In this book the eminent medical doctor tells how to get well and how to stay well, the drugless way. He was a thinker, a leader in thought, not a follower. He wrote:

"After years of wandering in the jungle of medical diagnosis—the usual guesswork of cause and effect and the worse-than-guesswork of treatment and becoming more confounded all the time—I resolved either to quit the profession or to find the cause of disease.

"My discovery of the truth that *toxemia* is the cause of all so-called diseases came about slowly, step by step, with many dangerous skids.

"That I have discovered the true cause of disease cannot be successfully disputed. This being true, my earnestness in presenting this great truth is justifiable.

"When I think back over my life and remember the struggle I had with myself in supplanting my old beliefs with the new—even doubting my own sanity—I then cannot be surprised at the opposition I have met and am meeting."

The writer of the Preface states: "His life was pre-eminently one of self-sacrifice and devotion to service, searching after truth with an indomitable will and with an intense fortitude to adhere to the truth when discovered. In his day Dr. Tilden's ideas received no support from the established medical profession, but brought the strongest of opposition and condemnation."

Times have not changed. These ideas are still calling forth extreme opposition, because they are utterly opposed to drugging as treatment.

"It was during the early years of his practice in Illinois that Dr. Tilden began to question the use of medicine to remedy illness. His extensive reading, especially of medical studies from European medical schools, and his own thinking led him to the conclusion that there should be some way to live so as not to build disease, and in this period his thoughts on toxemia began to formulate and materially develop. From the beginning of his practice in Denver the doctor used no medicine, but practiced his theory of clearing the body of toxic matter and then allowing inherent healing powers to restore health, teaching his patients how to live so as not to create a toxic condition and thus retain a healthy body free of disease."

Dr. Tilden wrote of his book: "What more can be asked of a health system than that it simplifies the cause of disease, making it understandable to all open-minded lay persons?

"*TOXEMIA EXPLAINED* does this very thing. If the reader will study this book as he/she must study a school book in order to understand it, he can learn what causes disease and knowing the cause, it will be an easy matter to avoid developing disease; but if imprudence brings on disease, he has the knowledge of how to overcome it."

"Disease is of man's own building, and one worse thing than the stupidity of buying a cure is to remain so ignorant as to believe in cures."

"The false theories of salvation and cures have built man into a mental mendicant when he could be the arbiter of his own salvation and certainly his own doctor instead of being a slave to a profession that has neither worked out its own salvation from disease nor discovered a single cure in all the age-long period of man's existence on earth.

"Every so-called disease is built within the mind and body by enervating habits. ... A fast, rest in bed and the giving-up of enervating habits, mental and physical, will allow nature to eliminate the accumulated toxin; then, if enervating habits are given up, and rational living habits adopted, health will come back to stay, if the one HEALED will stay put." This applies to any so-called disease.....

"Twenty-five years in which I used drugs and forty-three in which I have not used drugs should prove my conviction that drugs are unnecessary and in most cases injurious. ... Nature heals—nature can eliminate syphilis or any type of infection if all enervating habits are given up and a rational mode of living adopted. ...

"Germs and other so-called causes may be discovered in the course of pathological development, but they are accidental, coincidental or at most auxiliary." ...

"There is no hope that medical 'science' will ever be a science, for the whole structure is built around the idea that there is an entity—disease—that can be exorcised when the right drug is found." ...(the truth of the matter is that) "so-called disease is nature's effort to eliminate the toxin from the blood. All so-called diseases are crises of *toxemia* . ...Life as it is lived causes the people generally to be enervated. And when nerve energy drops below normal, the elimination of toxin—a natural product of metabolism—is checked and it is retained in the blood, bringing toxemia—the first, last, and only efficient cause of all so-called diseases."

"The amounts of harm done the army (and the people—Ed.) by vaccination and re-vaccination will never be known. No words can describe the harm that immunizing with vaccines and serums has done and is doing..."

In the section entitled "CRISES," Dr. Tilden writes: "According to the toxin philosophy, every so-called disease is a crisis of toxemia—which means that toxin has accumulated in the blood above the toleration point, and the crisis, the so-called disease—of whatever name—is a vicarious elimination. Nature is endeavoring to rid the body of toxin. Any treatment that obstructs this effort at elimination baffles nature in her effort at self-healing.

"Drugs, feeding, fear and keeping at work prevent elimination.

...The attending physician should know that every so-called disease is a complex of symptoms signifying a crisis of toxemia—nature's house cleaning. Nature can succeed admirably if not interfered with by vendors of poison, who are endeavoring to destroy an imaginary entity lurking somewhere in the system, which is mightily increased and intensified by the vendor's 'cures.' It is a real pleasure for the physician who knows that he cannot 'cure' anything to watch nature throw off all these symptoms by elimination if he is willing to do a little 'watchful waiting' and 'keep hands off.' ...

"Nature is not revengeful. Great suffering, chronic and fatal maladies are built by the incorrigibleness of patients and the well-meaning but belligerent efforts of the physicians who fight the imaginary foe without ceasing. The people are so saturated with the idea that disease must be fought to a finish that they are not satisfied with conservative treatment. Something must be done even if they pay for it with their lives, as millions do, every year. This willingness to die on the altar of medical superstition is one very great reason why no real improvement is made in fundamental medical science.

"**WHEN THE PEOPLE DEMAND <u>EDUCATION</u>—NOT MEDICATION, VACCINATION AND IMMUNIZATION—THEY WILL GET IT!**"

CONFESSIONS OF A MEDICAL HERETIC, Robert S. Mendelsohn, M.D., Contemporary Books, 1979.

Dr. Mendelsohn practiced medicine for thirty-four years before his recent passing. He was an effective writer and speaker, and had won the highest awards in his field. But he chose to be a critic of his profession, a medical heretic.

He believed that the greatest danger to your health is usually your own doctor. Modern medicine's methods, he stated, are rarely effective and in many instances are more dangerous than the diseases they are designed to diagnose and treat. He discussed iatrogenic diseases (originating with the physician or medicines).

In this book he tells why, if you're feeling fine, you should *not* have a physical examination, annually or otherwise. The effects of the exam may well be detrimental to your health, and the diagnosis, even if confirmed by laboratory tests, could very well be erroneous. In a recent nationwide examination of "high standard" laboratories, 50 percent failed.

Dr. Mendelsohn argues cogently that drugs are now being so overprescribed that more illnesses are being caused by their side effects—which doctors neglect to tell their patients about—than are being cured.

He discusses unnecessary surgery, birth at home versus the hospital, and so-called preventive medicine. He emphasizes that it is *your* health at stake and that *you* must finally make your own decisions regarding your medical treatment.

Dr. Mendelsohn also wrote *Malepractice: How Doctors Manipulate Women (1981), How to Have a Healthy Child in Spite of Your Doctor (1984)*, and contributed to *Dissent in Medicine: Nine Doctors Speak Out (1985)*.

In the last-named book, nine nationally known and highly-credentialed M. D.'s write. Robert S. Mendelsohn, George Crile, Samuel Epstein, Henry Heimlich, Alan Scott Levin, Edward R. Pinckney, David Spodick, Richard Moskowitz, and Gregory White each had lectured on a different topic at a conference of The New Medical Foundation. The lectures are reproduced in this book.

Lecture and chapter titles are as follows:

How Much Science is There is Modern Medicine—A Dissenting View; Treatment for Some Cancers—A Dissenting View; Environmental Issues in Medicine, A Dissenting View; Choking, Drowning and Resuscitation—Overcoming 25 years of Medical Errors; Corruption in American Medicine; The Accuracy of Medical Testing: A Dissenting View; Effectiveness of Treatment...A Cardiologist Dissents; Immunizations—A Dissenting View; and Hospital Births—A Dissenting View.

MEDICAL NEMESIS: The Expropriation of Health, by Ivan Illich. Pantheon Books, 1976.

Here is the essence of this book:

Modern medicine has reached the stage where it is itself a major threat to our health. This controversial book poses some basic questions not only about medicine but about the direction of modern society. Illich goes from a particular problem to a far more fundamental analysis. *Medical Nemesis* starts by focusing on a crisis that until now has been discussed primarily by doctors: the growth of iatrogenesis.

Iatrogenesis means illness caused by doctors, but Illich's book is not a narrow attack on the misapplication of medicine that has brought about so dramatic an increase in malpractice suits. It is instead a searching examination of what medicine really does, as opposed to the myth that has been built around it, and of the unfortunate dependence upon it that the modern world has developed. Carefully documenting his attack, Illich shows that major improvements in modern health have not come about primarily from improved medicine but from other factors outside of it (one is people improving their nutrition), and that the number of diseases that can be cured by medicine are nowhere near as great as the growing medical budgets would make us believe.

Modern medicine has not been able to heal many of the people who have come to depend on its "miracles." Some of the most expensive procedures have no proven effect whatsoever, or at best add only a few tortured years to the lives of patients who cannot really be cured. In short, medicine has not justified the faith with which people have turned over to doctors and to the medical system the fundamental decisions about their bodies and their lives.

Medical nemesis is bound to set in unless the autonomy of the individual is re-established. (This autonomy is the theme of our book, *They Conquered AIDS!*)

Ultimately, the danger we face is more than clinical iatrogenesis, more than the sum of malpractice, negligence, professional callousness, political mal-distribution, medically decreed disability, and all the consequences of medical trial and error. It is the expropriation of man's coping ability by a maintenance system that keeps him geared to the service of our industrial system.

Medical Nemesis was a best seller in several European countries and has set off, in France, Germany and Great Britain, a national debate on the implications of modern medicine that is long overdue.

The Lancet, prestigious journal of the British Medical Association, states: "*Medical Nemesis* is an important book. What gives Illich impact is an ability to provide a focus for increasing doubts. . . .There is indeed a strong case to answer."

New Scientist writes: "*Medical Nemesis* is disturbing and provocative. The urgency of the appeal and the passionate commitment to radical humanism shine through. The practice of medicine cannot stand still in a world which is currently undergoing exponential change."

WHAT YOUR DOCTOR DIDN'T LEARN IN MEDICAL SCHOOL (And What You Can Do About It!) by Stuart M. Berger, M.D. (Wm. Morrow & Co., N.Y. 1988.)

Dr. Berger courageously writes about the errors and failings of the medical system. "All of us, patient and practitioner alike, are caught in a vast, expensive, elaborate medical machine, one that very often works against our health and well-being. By being your own advocate, really understanding how the establishment works and making up yourself for what the medical machine lacks, you can turn it to your own advantage and beat the system."

This book is truly startling and extremely relevant to every American today. Stuart M. Berger, physician and best-selling author, is calling out: "WARNING! The medical system may be hazardous to your health!" He discusses the many unnecessary surgical procedures performed daily in the U.S.; the dangers of hospital-induced infection; the power of a profit-oriented insurance industry; how the training of today's doctors has all too often created specialized technicians who do not see their patients as unique human beings.

Dr. Berger tells of a family experience in 1976, while he was in his first year of medical school. It was a major medical foul-up, and his mother almost became a medical victim. She was about to be given poisonous chemotherapy. (In that period, doctors would take the patient to the brink of death with this treatment and then try to bring him back, not always successfully.) However, another doctor discovered that his mother did not have cancer, after all. He calls this wrenching experience "the excesses of medicine gone mad."

He began to see that our doctors, drugs and devices do not always create a happy ending. He is grateful for the skepticism implanted in him early in his career, and is acutely aware of the tragedies that often happen in hospitals. He sees many patients' handicaps and problems as entirely unnecessary; they occur because of what their doctors don't know.

As an impressionable medical student, he began questioning inside what he was learning to do and be. "I was beginning to ask what else I was being taught that they didn't really understand. Are we just learning to accept a whole system of medically-approved blind spots?"

His training was at the finest medical institutions—Tufts Medical School, the Harvard School of Public Health, etc. "We were learning immense amounts, but were we learning what we should? We were becoming doctors, to be sure, but were we becoming healers?"

He describes the brutal "rite of passage" of an intern. The young doctor goes to the ward for the first time and does not know what to do, but must do it for killing 36-hour stretches! The exhaustion he experiences is torture. Those years of residency hold agony and terror for the new intern. The system demands that the intern uses the patient as a human workbook! He is on his own. The years of medical school includes no training with patients. No wonder some serious, even fatal, mistakes occur in hospitals.

He quotes a faculty physician at John Hopkins Medical School: "We are entering a period in which a holistic conception of illness and healing is gaining ever wider acceptance."

He devotes an entire chapter to "The Miracles of Mental Medicine."

He and other innovative medical doctors are today exploring this exciting field.

Dr. Berger also devotes chapters to the "phantom" diseases—for example, candidiasis, which he discovered has its source in diet. But most doctors will not believe this, and give harmful drugs which only aggravate the problem. Also, patients are accused of being hypochondriacs—told by their doctors that their diseases are "imaginary," because the doctors do not understand the disease, or know how to overcome it!

Only reading this entire book will give you the whole story.

(This book is available on two cassette tapes from bookstores. Or call Dove Books on Tape. 800-345-9945.)

DIET FOR A NEW AMERICA: How Your Food Choices Affect Your Health, Happiness and the Future of Life on Earth, by John Robbins. Stillpoint, 1987.

Diet has been considered in many chapters of *They Conquered AIDS!* As the "Conquerors" lifted their consciousness, a vegetarian diet became part of their lifestyle in most cases. Anyone who wishes to attain better health and a higher consciousness should explore this diet, which is also a philosophy of "harmlessness" and a way of life.

There is a large vegetarian literature, and one of the best new books is entitled *Diet for a New America* by John Robbins. A fascinating aspect of this book is the author. He was heir to the ice cream fortune of the Baskin-Robbins company, but at age 20 was already enlightened in the New Age ideology. He turned his back on all he was born into—the wealth and the presidency-to-come of the large corporation.

This book is probably the most researched and complete book on the subject of the cruelty of factory farming, the environmental issues (cattle farming as destroying our forests, other land, and polluting our waters), the hunger issue (land can produce far more vegetarian food than flesh foods), and the health problems (meat as an markedly unhealthful food, from sick, diseased and chemical-ridden animals.) The topic deserves far more space than we can give here.

It is an eloquent book, this indictment of the meat, poultry, and dairy industries. John Robbins' *Diet for a New America* was nominated for a Pulitzer Prize in non-fiction in 1987. The author is the founder and president of EarthSave Foundation, whose theme is "human health, well-being and survival as being inextricably interwoven with the fate of all forms of life on Earth."

WHAT MUST I DO? Make Your Juicer Your Drug Store, by Dr. Laura Newman. Beneficial Books, a division of Benedict Lust Publications, 1970.

You have already read in *THEY CONQUERED AIDS!* two true life experiences concerning the powerful therapeutic effects of live vegetable juices. In the chapter by Russell John Carlton, the story of Mrs. Ferraro was told. Dying of leukemia, an eleventh-hour natural method was tried; it succeeded. She was given large quantities of freshly-squeezed carrot juice and no other food. She recovered. Russell also used fresh juices.

In the section by Dr. Gregory, "Why We Created This Book," he told of healing himself of a "staph" infection at age 15 by using chlorophyll and freshly squeezed vegetable juices from green, leafy vegetables. The condition was overcome quickly. Previously, weeks of antibiotics had only made the condition worse.

No one can consume enough raw vegetables in the amounts the body needs by chewing them. We are fortunate to live in a day when high-quality electric juicers for fruits and vegetables are available to us. These juicers are insufficiently appreciated and used, even by persons knowledgeable in natural health teachings.

This small volume by Dr. Laura Newman is a treasure. She covers a wide variety of topics, such as fatigue, elimination, circulatory and respiratory troubles, nerves, overweight, eye troubles, children's ailments, the teeth, etc. She devotes a chapter to the various juices she recommends, and gives the food values in each of the fruits and vegetables. Through study and practice for over 13 years, Dr. Newman compiled a wealth of knowledge.

Your juicer can not only become a source of healthful nourishment, but can become more valuable to you than a gold mine. Health is wealth.

John B. Lust, the publisher, also has books on this topic, entitled *Raw Juice Therapy* and *Drink Your Troubles Away.* Tree of Life Publications strongly recommends these books to all seekers of health the natural way.

A book should be written about carrots and carrot juice, alone. We know that Japanese pilots during World War II carried bottles of carrot juice around their necks, to partake of frequently. The reason is the powerful effect carrot juice has on vision.

Dr. Newman writes: "Carrots are fed to race horses, as they give lots of energy. Of course, a horse has a large stomach, but we can consume as many carrots as a horse can, if we throw away the roughage or cellulose and drink the raw juice which contains the valuable part of the carrot."

The book contains fascinating testimonies of many conditions corrected with live juices: hemorrhages, anemia, chronic fatigue, constipation, arthritis and rheumatism, etc. Equally or more important, the live juice program *prevents* disease, increases energy and nourishes the body with *pure liquid foods.*

Dr. Norman Walker, advocate of live juices who lived to 109, also wrote books on this subject: *Become Younger; Vibrant Health; Fresh Fruit and Vegetable Juices,* etc.

Carrots are an exceedingly rich source of Vitamin A, and a medium source of Vitamins B, C, and G. It is one of the most valuable of vegetables. Raw carrots contain nearly all the minerals and vitamins that are required by the human body. (U.S. Dept. of Agriculture.)

SPIRITUAL HEALING IN A SCIENTIFIC AGE, by Robert Peel. Harper & Row, 1987.

This inspiring book is an exploration of spiritual healing in a skeptical world. It is a provocative study, and addresses some of the most challenging spiritual questions of our times:

Is healing a science or an art? What is the place of spiritual healing in our scientific world? What place does prayer have in a technocratic society? Is spiritual healing a rational option today?

While based on the author's expert knowledge of Christian Science, this text offers a universality that appeals to many traditions and all seekers.

Most important, this book contains many personal testimonies— real experiences in spiritual healing from real lives.

One of them is by Friedrich Roselius of Lohhof, West Germany. He tells in detail of his long struggle with a serious case of eczema, and also a chronic thyroid ailment. Twenty-five years of medical treatment had failed to bring the slightest improvement. His mother confirms this fact, in a letter where she lists seventeen of the doctors who had treated her son over a 22-year period.

When Mr. Roselius heard of Christian Science, he began to study its textbook, *Science and Health.* He learned of his true relationship to God. The painful physical conditions vanished.

"It is our ignorance of God, the divine Principle, which produces apparent discord, and the right understanding of Him restores harmony." (Page 390, *Science and Health,* by Mary Baker Eddy.)

This testimony of spiritual healing is but one of many in the book by Robert Peel, and one of many thousands recorded elsewhere.

MARY EDDY BAKER, GOD'S GREAT SCIENTIST, in three volumes, by Helen M. Wright. (Mary Baker Eddy Institute, 2100 Third Ave., #2601, Seattle, WA 98121.)

This is the definitive biography written in our time. The trilogy explores Mary Baker Eddy's transformative first edition of *Science and Health* and of the remarkable woman who penned it. Its core teaching leads us out of materiality, translating human consciousness from matter back into Spirit. It breaks the hypnotic trance that buries us above-ground in matter beliefs, in bodies subject to sin, sickness, and death.

The way is shown us how to rethink ourselves into the truth of being, and learn that we are spiritual beings here and now, totally free. All must make the transition from a mortal sense of life to Life in and of Spirit. But first mankind must acknowledge this Science, study it, learn it.

We study the letter of Truth to gain the consciousness of Truth; then we find the structure of our consciousness conforming to the true spiritual reality. We become aware of Mary Baker Eddy's great yearning to free the human race "from the slavery of their own beliefs and from the educational systems...(that) hold the children of Israel (the whole human race) in bondage." (Science and Health, p. 226.)

BOOKS ON VACCINATION

Eleanor M. McBean, Ph.D., a former professor, has devoted a lifetime to research this vital subject. Her book *Vaccination Condemned* consists of 495 pages of eye-opening facts. It is available from Better Life Research, P. O. Box 42002, Los Angeles, CA 90042. (Dr. McBean's attempts to give copies to libraries met with refusal, because her books are not "medically approved.")

A review of the chapters' titles gives a good idea of the book's contents: Vaccination Condemned by All Competent Doctors; The Hazards of the Diphtheria Vaccine (DPT); Tetanus (Lockjaw) Caused Mainly by Vaccination; Warning Against the Measles Vaccine; How People Are Fooled by False Propaganda; Medically-Made Epidemics; Compulsory Vaccination is Illegal and Unconstitutional; How Vaccines Are Made; Crib Deaths Follow Vaccinations; Vaccination—a Leading Cause of TB; Whooping Cough and Mumps Vaccines, a Total Failure; Why Do Doctors Give Shots When They Know They Are Dangerous? Demand a Vaccination Guarantee (that it will not hurt you); How to Travel Abroad Without Vaccinations; Warning to Vaccination Promoters; The U.S. Has No Real Health Departments Nor Health Protection at Present.

Dr. McBean points out that many countries have banned vaccination, after learning from experience that <u>it does not protect from disease, but rather causes disease.</u> England has abolished compulsory vaccination, and the U.S. public should start waking up and move to influence their legislators to act in the same direction A second book on vaccination is *DON'T GET STUCK! The Case Against Vaccinations and Injections* by Hannah Allen. (Natural Hygiene Press, 1975.) The author is the current president of the American Natural Hygiene Society.

Mrs. Allen gives an interesting history of the vaccination practice, country by country, through hundreds of years. It started with a myth, about 1500 B.C. "Dhanwatari, the Vedic Father of Medicine, earliest known Hindu physician, was the first reported to have practiced inoculation for smallpox. In India and elsewhere, vaccination was a superstitious rite to (supposedly) placate and appease deities."

Alan Goldhamer, D.C., writes in the Introduction: "Hannah Allen mounts an effective challenge to one of conventional medicine's most 'sacred cows'—so-called immunization. She cogently advocates an end to compulsory inoculation and provides a wealth of documented information to stimulate the intelligent reader to re-examine assumptions concerning the risks and benefits of this practice, and to view this emotionally charged subject factually.

"A strong case is built supporting the self-healing, self-regulating nature of the human organism, and the pitfalls inherent in methodologies that obstruct natural processes."

One example Mrs. Allen gives of the harmfulness of inoculations follows: "VACCINES CAUSED SMALLPOX EPIDEMIC. Vaccination is the implantation of disease, and far from protecting against epidemics, it can actually cause and start them. Disease often attacks the vaccinated first. We have cited many instances of greater mass and individual susceptibility to disease after vaccination, such as the Cook County (Illinois) Hospital's immunization of one-half of their nursing staff against diphtheria. Diphtheria broke out soon afterward among the immunized cases, not the others. Also: within six years of the U.S. takeover of the Philippines and after 30,000,000 vaccinations, the Islands suffered more widespread smallpox than had ever occurred, and it was almost three times as fatal, with a death rate as high as 60-74 percent."

The vaccination practice is another glaring example of medical errors and superstitions that are perpetuated for hundreds of years, to mankind's detriment.

RELATED RECOMMENDED READING

FIT FOR LIFE. Harvey and Marilyn Diamond. Best seller; millions of copies sold. Based on Natural Hygiene principles.

LIVING HEALTH. Harvey and Marilyn Diamond. The in-depth follow-up to *Fit for Life*; goes beyond diet and explains how to design a total health program.

THE McDOUGALL PLAN. John McDougall, M.D. and Mary McDougall. The definitive vegetarian diet book. Renowned medical doctor documents the benefits.

YOU DON'T HAVE TO GET SICK! Jack Dunn Trop—one of the founders of the American Natural Hygiene Society (now 87 and still active).

THE FRUITARIAN SYSTEM OF HEALING. O.L.M. Abramowski, M.D.

LIVING LIFE TO LIVE IT LONGER. Herbert M. Shelton. He carried on Dr. Tilden's work and helped establish Natural Hygiene as a strong movement.

THE GREATEST HEALTH DISCOVERY—NATURAL HYGIENE, and Its Evolution, Past, Present & Future. From the works of the movement's 19th century pioneers. Ten medical doctors were the leaders of the early Natural Hygiene movement. They found their practices to be a wrong approach to health care and were led to discover that there are natural laws which govern human life that, when applied, can both maintain and recover health.

SUPERIOR NUTRITION. Herbert M. Shelton.

SUNLIGHT COULD SAVE YOUR LIFE. Zane R. Kime, M.D. This best seller of 1980 on sun therapy or heliotherapy reveals how you can lower your cholesterol, blood pressure, and blood sugar; how you can increase your endurance, sex hormones, and resistance to infection. Includes a crucial sunbather's diet.

BOOKS ON FASTING

FASTING CAN SAVE YOUR LIFE. Herbert M. Shelton. (500,000 copies sold.) "Here is an amazing new approach to health and happiness. It does not discuss theories; it deals with facts. . .Discover how your body has remarkable regenerative powers!"

Dr. Shelton's dedication is: "To the millions of sufferers who are agonizing throughout their lives in search of health and not knowing where or how to find it. My firm conviction is born of years of practical experience in the application of fasting to the problems of health. It is that fasting and a *Hygienic* way of life will lead to vigorous health."

THE SCIENCE AND FINE ART OF FASTING. Herbert M. Shelton

FASTING FOR THE HEALTH OF IT. Oswald/Shelton

THE FASTING CURE. Upton Sinclair

FASTING FOR HEALTH AND LONG LIFE. Hereward Carrington, Ph.D.

THERAPEUTIC FASTING. Arnold De Vries

SCIENTIFIC FASTING. Linda B. Hazzard, D.O.

HOW TO KEEP SLIM, HEALTHY, & YOUNG WITH JUICE FASTING. Paavo Airola, N.D., Ph.D.

FASTING: Fastest Way to Super Health and Rejuvenation. Your First Fast— What to Expect. Hannah Allen.

RATIONAL FASTING for Physical, Mental & Spiritual Rejuvenation. Prof. Arnold Ehret.

Many of these books are available from Vegetarian Society, Inc., P. O. Box 126, Joshua Tree, CA 92252

Books by N. W. Walker, D.Sc., Ph.D.

This remarkable man pioneered juice therapy and colonic irrigations, for internal cleanliness. He lived to 109, productive (writing, gardening) until the very end of his life.

His books:

BECOME YOUNGER   COLON HEALTH: Key to a Vibrant Life   FRESH VEGETABLE AND FRUIT JUICES   DIET AND SALAD SUGGESTIONS WATER CAN UNDERMINE YOUR HEALTH   NATURAL WEIGHT CONTROL

Dr. Walker also created three charts: *Colon Therapy, The Endocrine Gland,* and *Foot Relaxation.* Health product stores have his works or can order them for you.

BOOKS SUGGESTED BY THE "CONQUERORS" OR MENTIONED BY THE AUTHORS

Abrahamson, E. M., and Pezet, A. W. *Body, Mind & Sugar*. New York: Holt, Rinehart and Winston, 1951.

Airola, Paavo. *How to Keep Slim, Healthy and Young with Juice Fasting*. Phoenix: Health Plus, 1971.

Anonymous. *A Course in Miracles*. Tiburon, CA: The Foundation for Inner Peace, 1975.

Anonymous. *The Lost Books of the Bible and The Forgotten Books of Eden*. New American Library, 1948.

Appleton, Nancy. *Lick the Sugar Habit*. New York: Warner Books, 1985.

Arms, Suzanne. *Immaculate Deception—A New Look at Women and Childbirth*. New York: Bantam Books, 1977.

Bach, Richard. *Illusions: The Adventures of a Reluctant Messiah*. New York: Delacorte, 1977. New York, NY: Dell, 1979.

Berger, Stuart M. *What Your Doctor Didn't Learn in Medical School*. New York: Morrow & Co., 1988.

Bible, The Holy.

Cantwell, Alan, Jr. *AIDS: The Mystery and the Solution*. Los Angeles: Aries Rising Press, (Rev.) 1986.

_____.*AIDS and the Doctors of Death*. Same publisher, 1988.

Cousins, Norman. *Anatomy of an Illness as Perceived by the Patient*. New York: Bantam Books/Norton, 1979.

_____.*The Healing Heart, Antidote to Panic*. W. W. Norton, 1983.

Dufty, William. *Sugar Blues*. New York: Warner Books, 1975.

Eddy, Mary Baker. *Science and Health with Key to the Scriptures*. Boston: The Christian Science Publishing Society.

_____.*Miscellaneous Writings*. Same publisher.

_____.*Prose Works*. Same publisher.

Feingold, Ben. *Why Your Child is Hyperactive*. New York: Random House, 1975.

Gawain, Shakti. *Creative Visualization*. New York: Bantam Books, 1978.

Gregory, Scott & Leonardo, Bianca. *Conquering AIDS Now!* Santa Monica: Tree of Life Publications, 1986. New York: Warner Books, 1987.

Haich, Elisabeth. *Initiation*. Palo Alto: Seed Center, 1974.

Harrison, John. *Love Your Disease—It's Keeping You Healthy.* London: Angus and Robertson Publishers.

Hay, Louise L. *You Can Heal Your Life.* Santa Monica: Hay House, 1984.

_____ .*AIDS: A Positive Approach.* Same Publisher, 1987.

Holmes, Ernest. *A New Design for Living.* Englewood Cliffs: Prentice-Hall, 1983.

_____ .*This Thing Called Life.* New York: Dodd-Mead, 1947.

_____ .*This Thing Called You.* New York: Dodd-Mead, 1948.

Kelder, Peter. *Ancient Secret of the Fountain of Youth.* (Rev. ed.) Gig Harbor, WA: Harbor Press, 1986.

Kushi, Michio. *Crime & Diet: The Macrobiotic Approach.* Japan Publications, USA, 1987.

Leonard, Ann. *The Five Elements of Rebirthing.* 1986.

Leonard, Jim and Laut, Phil. *Rebirthing — The Science of Enjoying All of Your Life.* Cincinnati: Trinity Press, 1983.

Leonardo, Bianca. *Deep Thoughts on War and Peace and Other Essays on the Vegetarian Way of Life.* Tree of Life Publications, 1986.

_____ . *Cancer & Other Diseases Caused by Meat Consumption,* same publisher, 1986

Matthews-Simonton, Stephanie and Simonton, O. Carl. *Getting Well Again.* New York: Bantam, 1980.

Nelson, Ruby. *The Door of Everything.* Marina Del Rey: De Vorss & Co., 1963.

Notovitch, Nicholas. *The Unknown Life of Jesus Christ.* Tree of Life Publications, 1980.

Pearsall, Paul. *Superimmunity.* Los Angeles: J.P. Tarcher, 1987.

Rajneesh, Bhagwan S. *The Book of Wisdom* Vol. 2. Boulder: Chidvilas Foundation, 1984.

Ray, Sondra. *Celebration of Breath.* Berkeley: Celestial Arts, 1983.

_____ .*Loving Relationships.* Berkeley: Celestial Arts, 1980.

Robbins, John. *Diet for a New America.* Walpole, NH: Stillpoint, 1987

Robinson, James M. *The Nag Hammadi Library.* New York: Harper & Row, 1977.

Rodale, J. I. *Natural Health, Sugar and the Criminal Mind.* Pyramid Books, 1968.

Rossi, Ernest. *The Psychobiology of Mind-Body-Healing.* New York: W. W. Norton & Co., 1988.

Shelton, Herbert M. *Fasting Can Save Your Life.* Bridgeport, CT: Natural Hygiene Press, 1981.

____ .*Fasting for Renewal of Life.* Chicago: Natural Hygiene Press, 1974.

____ .*The Science and Fine Art of Fasting.* Chicago: Natural Hygiene Press, 1978.

Shilts, Randy. *And The Band Played On: Politics, People, and the AIDS Epidemic.* New York: St. Martin's Press, 1987.

Siegel, Bernie S., *Love, Medicine & Miracles.* New York: Harper & Row, 1986.

Smyly, Barbara and Glen. *All in the Name of Love.* Land O' Lakes, FL: Alivening Publications, 1986.

Spalding, Baird T. *The Life and Teachings of the Masters of the Far East,* 5 volumes. Marina del Rey, CA: De Vorss & Co., 1924.

Szekely, Edmond B., translator. *The Essene Gospel of Peace.* Cartago, Costa Rica: International Biogenic Society, 1931.

Trimarchi, Angelo. *AIDS: Don't Die of Ignorance.* From the Natural Hygiene viewpoint. Translated into English from Italian. Available from Tree of Life Publications; see address below.

Ullman, Dana. *Homeopathy: Twenty-First Century Medicine.* Berkeley: North Atlantic, 1988.

Yudkin, John. *Sweet and Dangerous.* New York: Bantam Books, 1972.

More True Life Adventures by AIDS Conquerors are welcome. Please write the publishers. See address in box below. ---

New Views in Healing & AIDS Update

A Newsletter about Health, Hope, and Humanity
Ask for Brochure
Tree of Life Publications
255 N. El Cielo Rd., # 126
Palm Springs, CA 92262

358 • THEY CONQUERED AIDS!

Diet for a New America, 347
Diet, 113, 119, 254, 277, 294
Dis-ease, 188
Dissatisfied Parents Together, 330
Dissent in Medicine: Nine Doctors Speak Out, 344
Don't Get Stuck! The Case Against Vaccination, 351
Drink Your Troubles Away, 348
Drugs, 57-58
Drugs as sorcery, 317
Drugs, recreational, 262
Drugs, side effects, 42, 219
Dyspnea, 314
EarthSave Foundation, 347
Eddy, Mary Baker, 187, 208, 303
"Edge" magazine, 97
Educating oneself, 189, 211
Einstein, Albert, 226
ELISA Test, 105, 155, 200, 274
Emergence, Int., 304
Emotional states, 206
Enthusiasm, 262
Essene Gospel of Peace, 88
Essentials of health, seven, 317
Fasting, 81-82, 100, 298-300, 307
Fasting books, 100, 352-353
Fear, 56, 118, 136, 138-139, 257, 265, 295
Ferraro, Mrs., 101, 348
Fire walk, 290
Fisher, Barbara Loe, 330-31
Fit for Life, 351
Five Rites, 233, 247-49
Flagyl, 288
Food, natural, 142, 158
Food: pure in the plant kingdom vs. flesh foods, 190-191
Freedom of choice in health, 309, 328
Friendships, 214, 235
Fruitarian System of Healing, 352
Galen, 39
Gallo, Robert, M.D., x
Gawain, Shakti, 119
Gay Men's Health Crisis, 120
Gay Metaphysical-Spiritual Assn., 152,159
"Gay Plague," 140
Getting Well Again, 236, 291
Giving and receiving, 187
God, xiv, 94-95,189, 235-36, 238, 264, 294-95, 312
God as Love, 145, 159, 177
Goldhamer, Alan, D.C., 351
Gottlieb, Dr. Michael, 230
Graham, Dr. Mateel, 265
Grand mal seizures, 203

Greatest Health Discovery, 352
"Greer, Steven," 262-270
Grief, 67, 140
Griggs, Tommy, 149-163
Group therapy, 266
Guided Imagery and Music, 228-29
Guilt, 308
Hahneman, Samuel, 40
Haiti, x
Hampton, John, 300-301
Harbor General Hospital, 154
Hay, Louise, 63-64, 195, 289
"Healing AIDS," newsletter, 325
Healing modes, 35-48
Health knowledge, 308, 310
Health quotations, 337
Hepatitis, 130, 132, 137, 232,263
Hepatitis B vaccine trials, ix
Herbal tea, 80-1
Herbs, 36,211,255,276-7
Himalayan International Inst. of Yoga, 164
Hippocrates, 37-39, 41, 282
HIV (AIDS virus), ix
Holistic & spiritual techniques, 168, 220-221
Holistic healing, 53-54, 82, 95-96, 184, 194, 205, 210, 218, 239, 307, 311-12, 315
Holmes, Dr. Ernest: books by, 168, 176
Holmes, Oliver Wendell, 57,
Homeopathy, 40-42
Homeopathy: Medicine for the 21st Century, 42
Homosexual community, xiv
How to Get Free Press, 331
How to Have a Healthy Child in Spite of Your Doctor, 344
How to Keep Slim, Healthy and Young with Juice Fasting, 299
Humor, 239
Hygeia, goddess of health, 46, 100
Hygeia Health Retreat, 299
Illich, Ivan, 344-45
Immaculate Deception—A New Look at Women & Childbirth, 39-40
Immuno-suppressive drugs, legal, 257
Interferon, 263
Intuition, 120
"J.H.," 301-302
James, William, 33
John David Learning Institute, 237
Johnson, Douglas, 166-181
Judgement, 203, 308-309
Juices, 100-101
Kaposi's sarcoma (KS), xi, xii, 55-56, 128-29, 130-31, 169, 254, 263, 302
Khalil, Mina, 276
Kierson, Ellie, 186, 215, 225-29